To Listen,

To Comfort,

To Care

To Listen,
To Comfort,
To Care:
Reflections
on Death
and Dying

Barbara Backer, RN, DSW
Associate Professor, Division of Nursing
Lehman College, City University of New York
Bronx, New York

Natalie Hannon, PhD
Director of Training and Staff Development
Bronx-Lebanon Hospital Center
Bronx, New York

Joan Young Gregg, PhD
Professor, New York City Technical College
City University of New York
New York, New York

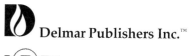
Delmar Publishers Inc.™
I͟T͟P™

12-94

Notice to the Reader

Publisher does not warrant or guarantee any of the products described herein or perform any independent analysis in connection with any of the product information contained herein. Publisher does not assume, and expressly disclaims, any obligation to obtain and include information other than that provided to it by the manufacturer.

The reader is expressly warned to consider and adopt all safety precautions that might be indicated by the activities described herein and to avoid all potential hazards. By following the instructions contained herein, the reader willingly assumes all risks in connection with such instructions.

The publisher makes no representations or warranties of any kind, including but not limited to, the warranties of fitness for particular purpose or merchantability, nor are any such representations implied with respect to the material set forth herein, and the publisher takes no responsibility with respect to such material. The publisher shall not be liable for any special, consequential or exemplary damages resulting, in whole or in part, from the readers' use of, or reliance upon, this material.

Cover Design: J² Designs

Delmar staff:
Publisher: David C. Gordon
Senior Acquisitions Editor: Bill Burgower
Assistant Editor: Debra M. Flis
Project Editor: Danya M. Plotsky
Production Coordinator: Barbara A. Bullock
Art and Design Coordinators: Megan K. DeSantis
Timothy J. Conners

For information, address

Delmar Publishers Inc.
3 Columbia Circle, Box 15015
Albany, NY 12212-5015

Copyright © 1994 by Delmar Publishers Inc.

The trademark ITP is used under license.

Printed in the United States of America
Published simultaneously in Canada
by Nelson Canada,
a division of The Thomson Corporation

1 2 3 4 5 6 7 8 9 10 XXX 00 99 98 97 96 95 94

Library of Congress Cataloging-in-Publication Data

Backer, Barbara A.
    To listen, to comfort, to care : reflections on death and dying /
Barbara Backer, Natalie Hannon, Joan Young Gregg.
      p.   cm. — (Real nursing series)
    Includes index.
    ISBN 0-8273-6178-5
    1. Nursing—Psychological aspects. 2. Terminal care. I. Hannon,
Natalie. II. Gregg, Joan Young. III. Title. IV. Series.
    [DNLM: 1. Death. 2. Attitude to Death. 3. Terminal Care—
psychology. 4. Nursing care—psychology. BF 789.D4 B126t 1993]
RT87.T45B33 1993
362 1'75'024613—dc20
DNLM/DLC
for Library of Congress
                                   93-26362
                                      CIP

RealNursing Series
Alice M. Stein, MA, RN, Series Editor
Medical College of Pennsylvania

HEALING YOURSELF: A NURSE'S GUIDE TO SELF-CARE AND RENEWAL
COMMUNICATION AND IMAGE IN NURSING
FEAR AND AIDS/HIV: EMPATHY AND COMMUNICATION
SEXUAL HEALTH: A NURSE'S GUIDE
20 LEGAL PITFALLS FOR NURSES TO AVOID
TO LISTEN, TO COMFORT, TO CARE: REFLECTIONS ON DEATH AND DYING
THE NURSE AS HEALER
MEDICATION ERRORS: THE NURSING EXPERIENCE

FUTURE TITLES:

CRITICAL BUSINESS SKILLS FOR NURSES
HEALING ALCOHOL AND SUBSTANCE ABUSE
ETHICAL DILEMMAS IN NURSING
WAR STORIES: DIFFICULT NURSING DECISIONS
THE FEMINIST NURSE
THE GAY AND LESBIAN NURSE
INTERVENTIONS IN EVERYDAY NURSING EMERGENCIES
HEALING RACISM IN NURSING

EAGLE POEM
by Joy Harjo

To pray you open your whole self
To sky, to earth, to sun, to moon
To one whole voice that is you.
And know there is more
That you can't see, can't hear
Can't know except in moments
Steadily growing, and in languages
That aren't always sound but other
Circles of motion.
Like eagle that Sunday morning
Over Salt River. Circled in blue sky
In wind, swept our hearts clean
With sacred wings.
We see you, see ourselves and know
That we must take the utmost care
And kindness in all things.
Breathe in, knowing we are made of
All this, and breathe, knowing
We are truly blessed because we
Were born, and die soon, within a
True circle of motion,
Like eagle rounding out the morning
Inside us.
We pray that it will be done
In beauty.
In beauty.

Reprinted from *In Mad Love & War* © 1990 by Joy Harjo, Wesleyan University Press.
By permission of University Press of New England.

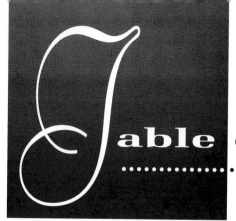

Table of Contents

PREFACE ■ xiii

CHAPTER 1 ■ 1
DEATH IN AMERICAN SOCIETY

Changing Mortality Patterns 5
American Values 6
Institutionalization of Dying 6
Death in Society Today 7

CHAPTER 2 ■ 11
DEATH AND THE PROCESS OF DYING

Developmental Influences on Perceptions of Death 13
Fear of Death and Dying, and Death Anxiety 16
Dying as a Process 18
Stigma and the Dying Person 20
Talking with People about Their Dying 23
Coping with Death and Dying 25

CHAPTER 3 ■ 29
THE HELPING PROFESSIONS AND
THE TERMINALLY ILL

Nurses 31
Physicians 38
Communication between Nurses and Physicians 42

CHAPTER 4 ■ 47
HOSPITALS AND DYING PATIENTS

A History of Hospital Care 49
Role Expectations 53
Disclosing Information to Patients 56
Influences on Patient Care 58
Alternatives to Hospital Care 60

CHAPTER 5 ▪ 63
HOSPICE CARE AND PAIN MANAGEMENT

History of the Hospice 65
Hospice Care in the United States 67
Pain Management 69
The Institutional Setting and Pain Management 76

CHAPTER 6 ▪ 79
CHILDREN AND DEATH

Children's Concepts of Death 81
Talking with Children about Death and Dying 84
Caregivers and Terminally Ill Children 87
Families and Terminally Ill Children 89
Home Care for Dying Children 94
The Death of an Infant 96

CHAPTER 7 ▪ 99
LIVING WITH AIDS
(BY KATHLEEN M. NOKES)

Understanding HIV Disease 101
The Face of Persons with AIDS 104
Health Care Concerns of Persons with AIDS 105
Concerns of Families and Loved Ones 109
Concerns of Health Care Providers 112
Ethical Issues 115

CHAPTER 8 ▪ 119
ETHICAL AND LEGAL ISSUES

The Definition of Death 121
The Right to Refuse Treatment 124
Euthanasia 127

CHAPTER 9 ▪ 133
SUICIDE

Who Attempts or Commits Suicide? 135
Theories of Suicide 139
Suicide Prevention 144
The Impact of Suicide on Survivors 148
The Health Care Professional's Response to Suicide 149

CHAPTER 10 ■ 151
GRIEF AND BEREAVEMENT

Grief 153
The Symptomatology of Grief and Bereavement 156
Pathological Grief Reactions 157
Anticipatory Grief 159
Parents' Grief 161
Role Changes after the Death of a Spouse 162
Caregivers' Roles with the Bereaved 164

CHAPTER 11 ■ 167
DEATH FROM A CROSS-CULTURAL PERSPECTIVE (BY SERENA NANDA)

Beliefs about the Afterlife 169
Attitudes Toward Pain, Dying, and Death 171
Grief Reactions: Common Experiences 172
The Rituals of Death: Funerals and Mourning 176

INDEX ■ 183

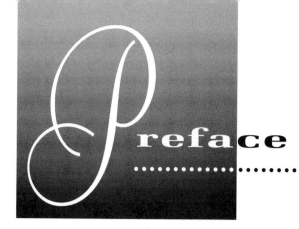

Preface

To listen, to comfort, and to care are behaviors and feelings that many people want to express, to give, and to experience when faced with grief, death, and dying. However, in American culture and in today's high-tech medical system, understanding and care are not as valued as efficiency and cost-effectiveness. Health care professionals are continually challenged to create for and with their patients a way of experiencing death and grieving that supports the quality, uniqueness, and dignity of each person's life.

This book is an adaptation of our text, *Death and Dying: Understanding and Care*, 2nd edition; Joan Gregg has joined us as editor. The concept of caring is inherent in both books, and continues to be used here to connote enabling and supporting. The dying person's feelings and thoughts, and those of their significant others, are integral and acknowledged components of this concept of care. Confronting death, or coping with the death of a loved one encompasses a complex set of human behaviors and feelings which many people seek within the self, the family, culture, and religion. A caregiver, friend, or relative providing care is challenged to recognize these complexities, and to understand and support the person who is coping with death and dying. Our reflections on death and dying include the increasing cultural diversity of Americans and the importance of recognizing how the experience of death and dying and loss can be lived in so many different ways. To listen then, becomes a valued component of care and comfort.

Many people have supported and encouraged us in developing this book. We would like to acknowledge Debra Flis, assistant editor, for her accessibility and competence in manuscript preparation, Elayne Rinn for her skill and patience in typing, and Bill Burgower for his guidance as senior administrative editor. We would also like to express our gratitude and appreciation to our students and patients, who have been continuing sources of motivation and enrichment.

Barbara A. Backer
Natalie Hannon
Joan Young Gregg

Chapter 1

Death in American Society

Try talking about dying and death at a party. Watch people's reactions: many will move away; some will joke about the subject; others may simply say, "I don't want to talk about such a morbid topic." But there will also be a group of people fascinated by the subject, and a lively conversation may ensue. While most people do not want to deal with the fact that sooner or later we all will die, there is in American society an increasing realization that dealing with the subject of death allows people to live their lives more fully.

Thanatologists, specialists who study the various aspects of death and dying, have called the United States a death-denying society. Yet this is too simple. While most Americans may not wish to talk about death and dying at a party, nevertheless Elisabeth Kübler-Ross's book *On Death and Dying* and Derek Humphrey's *Final Exit*, a book on how to commit suicide, were best-sellers among trade paperbacks. And although most of us do not experience the death of a loved one until adulthood, many children see death portrayed on television practically every night. It is probably more accurate to say that instead of denying death, Americans are ambivalent in their feelings about death and dying.

Attitudes and feelings toward death and dying have changed over time. The French scholar Phillippe Aries (Note 1) traced the cultural attitudes toward death since the Middle Ages. The traditional attitude toward death was one of resignation and acceptance. In the ancient past, death and life were considered to exist simultaneously. Death was both "familiar and near, evoking no great fear or awe." During the Middle Ages, with the growing importance of religion and the effects of the Black Death, people not only resigned themselves to the deaths of others but also accepted their own dying and death.

One could not be isolated from death. In the fourteenth century, for example, the Black Death was said to have killed more than 25% of the population of Europe; later, in 1603, one-fifth of the population of London was killed by the plague. As the famous diarist Samuel Pepys recorded in his journal:

June 15th, 1665. The Towne grows very sickly, and people to be afeard of it; there dying this last week of plague 112, from 43 the week before.

August 10th, 1665. By and by to the office, where we sat all the morning; in great trouble to see the Bill this week rise so high, to above 4,000 in all, and of them above 3,000 of the plague. . . . The town growing so unhealthy, that a man cannot depend upon living two days to an end.

September 20th, 1665. But, Lord! what a sad time it is to see no boats upon the River; and grass grows all up and down White Hall court, and nobody but poor wretched in the streets! And, which is worst of all, the Duke showed us the number of the plague this week, brought in the last night from the Lord Mayor; that it is encreased from about 600 more than the last, which is quite contrary to all our hopes and expectations, from the coldness of the late season. For the whole general number is 8,297, and of them the plague 7,165 (Pepys, Note 2).

With the ascendance of Catholicism and then Protestantism, death came to be viewed as a form of justice. To have a good life after death, it was imperative for the dying person to have behaved well in life. People had to prepare to meet their maker in the proper manner. True salvation could only be found if all mortal passions were renounced; humanity was to concentrate only on God.

Beginning in the eighteenth century, people again became concerned with the death of others, which Aries calls "Thy Death." Rather than being viewed as a part of life, death was seen as a break with life. Death was both frightening and fascinating, but it was also romanticized; the death of another person became more fearful than one's own death. Mourning was exaggerated, and elaborate memorials and monuments were built for the dead. In the American colonies, for example, funerals were extravagant social gatherings on which hundreds of pounds were spent to mark the death of an individual.

In the mid-nineteenth century, the period of "Forbidden Death" began. Death became a technological phenomenon. Death no longer occurred in the home, but in the hospital, which eliminated any ceremony between the family and the dying person. In addition, funerals began to be held at specialized "parlors," not in the home. Death was no longer a part of everyday life. A silence fell over the subject, and death was viewed, like sex, as something disgusting and unsuitable for acknowledgment or discussion.

Today, however, people are no longer silent on the subject of death. Since the 1960s, there has been a great deal of talk about death. With the writings of Kübler-Ross, the hospice movement, the raising of many ethical issues concerning death, AIDS, and the death education movement, our society has moved from the denial of death to the "containment of death." The prolongation of life is highly valued, and the chief concern now is with controlling and managing death and dying. Although there might seem to be a contradiction between America's traditional orientation toward denying death and the recent emphasis on death awareness, in fact these two attitudes can be easily reconciled. In order to understand why society tries to "contain" death, such factors as changing mortality patterns, American values, and the institutionalization of dying must be taken into account.

CHANGING MORTALITY PATTERNS

With the change from a preindustrial to an industrial society, mortality patterns changed from uncontrolled to controlled. Uncontrolled mortality had three patterns: mortality was high, it fluctuated over short periods, and it varied widely at any point in time. With controlled mortality, however, the opposite conditions prevail: mortality is low and does not fluctuate widely either over time or geographic area.

In the seventeenth century, the average life expectancy ranged from 20 to 40 years, and mortality rates could be as high as 400 per 1000 population during times of famine and epidemics. In the eighteenth century, there were epidemics of smallpox, cholera, and typhus. For instance, 25% of the population of France was killed, crippled, or disfigured by smallpox. Under this uncontrolled mortality, death was both random and constantly present. Thus society had to incorporate death into the everyday values and structures.

Today, under conditions of controlled mortality, the average life expectancy in the United States is 75 years of age. The death rate is 8.5 per 1,000 population. Furthermore, this death rate has hardly fluctuated for the past 20 years. In addition, controlled mortality has changed the demographics of those who are dying. Prior to controlled mortality, the very young and the middle-aged were most likely to die. Even one of the most privileged groups in preindustrial society, the British aristocracy, had an infant mortality rate of 200 per 1,000 live births. In those days, if you were able to survive beyond infancy, you were likely to die in the middle of adulthood, or your spouse was. Death had to be confronted. In contrast, today in the United States the infant mortality rate is approximately 9.1 per 1,000 live births (although the infant mortality rate for African-Americans is almost double the rate for whites). Furthermore, it is the elderly who are most likely to die. Therefore, many Americans do not consider it necessary to incorporate an awareness of death into their lives before they are old. Our expectation is that we will have many years to live, in which to accomplish and to achieve our goals. Thus, we spend a great deal of money and energy on research and therapies aimed at curing disease and extending life. Our culture fosters future-oriented attitudes of planning, saving, and deferred gratification. In America, the concentration is on prolonging life, not on the relevance of death.

AMERICAN VALUES

Implicit in American values are the notions of innovation, efficiency, and progress. Since science and technology are central in our value system, death is approached in this light. Through science and technology, Americans can maintain the illusion of conquering death, an illusion strengthened by the fact that Americans' life span has increased by more than 20 years since 1900. Today, we die of the diseases of old age: heart disease, cancer, and stroke cause more than 60% of the deaths in this country.

The American emphasis on using science and technology to control death is symbolized by the development of a new word, *prolongevity*, which implies that we have the ability to prolong our lives. Americans rely more than ever on the skill of doctors, on diet, and on medicaments, to postpone death. Our need to control death is also evidenced, more recently, by our reactions to AIDS. AIDS has upset American ideas about containing death. Although we know that AIDS is caused by a virus, we cannot predict the course of the virus, nor can we kill it. AIDS is a disease of the young and middle-aged, and we do not seem to be able to control its spread. AIDS presents us with the reality that death ultimately denies rational analysis.

Another value important in American society is happiness. Our advertising industry, with its emphasis on youth, has contributed to the belief that we must be happy. Dying and death interfere with happiness, and we do not want to accept this interference. As the historian Arnold Toynbee said: "For Americans, death is un-American, and an affront to every citizen's inalienable right to life, liberty and the pursuit of happiness" (Toynbee, Note 3).

INSTITUTIONALIZATION OF DYING

With our control over mortality and our belief that death can be avoided, dying has become institutionalized. No longer do most people die at home with their families; almost 80% of Americans die in hospitals.

Since most people now die in hospitals, dying has become invisible. Hospitals view themselves as places that cure, not care for, the dying. Thus, there is very little room for the dying or for grieving families in such institutions.

In fact, hospitals attempt to make the dying and the dead invisible. Elisabeth Kübler-Ross recounts how, when she asked to interview a dying patient for a seminar she was giving, there were, suddenly, no dying patients in that hospital. This death denial in American hospitals is also illustrated by a passage in a current text on hospital administration that suggests that the best place for a hospital morgue is on the ground floor, in an area inaccessible to the general public, with an exit leading onto a private, concealed loading platform. Another example of death denial occurred in the planning of the renovation of a major medical center in New York City where no space was allocated for the morgue. Only at the medical center's renovation was a morgue built in, located in a very inconvenient area of the hospital.

Our institutionalized dying presents a sharp contrast to the following account of a woman dying in the nineteenth century: "Mother Drinkwater was critically ill, but some of her family realized the seriousness of her condition. Never having been to a hospital, and without recent contact with a physician, she remained in bed while the rest of the family carried out their regular activities. They took turns caring for her as best they could. One night while Mary was sitting up with her, Mother Drinkwater 'seemed to die in her sleep.' Her husband, son and daughter were asleep in other parts of the house" (Rosenblatt, Note 4).

Today, with hospices, there is an attempt to move dying back into the home. There are more than 1,700 hospices in the United States, and the primary type of hospice care involves home care. Hospices care not just for the dying patient, but for the patient and the family. It is an attempt to bring the family back into the process of dying and to make dying visible again.

DEATH IN SOCIETY TODAY

In our society, no one ever dies. We "pass on," or we "rest in peace"; our pets are "put to sleep." Even in hospitals patients do not die, they expire. Our funeral practices are such that we attempt to make the corpse look as alive as possible, even using special garments and cosmetics. We are also concerned with the comfort of the body within the casket.

Death is distorted in the media as well, where it is either romanticized or depicted as violent. Movies show dying people closing their eyes upon death, although in fact most people die with their eyes open. Violent death is ubiquitous on television and in the movies. A typical adolescent television viewer has witnessed some 18,000 homicides on the screen. These are media myths, however, for most of us will not die either with a smile on our faces and holding hands with our loved ones, or in the violent fashion portrayed in police stories.

These contradictory and ambiguous attitudes toward death and dying have led us into a number of problematic areas. How is a person supposed to act when dying? Since those who are dying are generally elderly and isolated in hospitals, we have not seen how people act in this role. Many of us today are without beliefs about the meaning of death. We have little experience in dealing with death or dying in our families, and we are not taught as children about the proper behaviors for dealing with the dying and the bereaved. As adults, then, we find it difficult to face either our own death or the deaths of others. Even hospital personnel have trouble caring for the dying properly.

Along with these problems, however, come potential solutions: new roles can be developed in which the dying can, if they so choose, talk about their feelings and their dying; new organizations can be designed, such as the hospices, where the care and comfort of the terminally ill are the primary goals; and new meanings for death can be constructed.

Throughout the 1970s and 1980s in the United States, people began to talk about death and dying. Americans have become concerned about the various ethical and practical issues that arise from dealing with death as a technological phenomenon, perhaps because we are becoming an older society. In 2020, the aged are expected to make up almost 16% of the American population. This means that dying is becoming more relevant to more people.

Another answer to the problem of learning to deal with death lies in the work of two women: Dr. Kübler-Ross and Dr. Cicely Saunders. The publication of Kübler-Ross's book *On Death and Dying* exposed readers to issues in the health care delivery system and crystallized not only the problem of the dying patient but also the difficulty faced by those whose task it is to deal with the hidden issues of death in a public setting. With the work of Cicely Saunders, the founder of the modern hospice movement, the British and American societies have been led toward a more humane way of treating the dying. The hospice movement has forced hospitals to look at how the dying were being treated, and has led to an interest in caring for the dying with respect and dignity, and with concern for their pain.

Still another basis for our new concern with death and dying lies in the development of advanced technologies that can prolong the life of those whose quality of life has severely diminished. The development of technology that allows us to save lives by such means as organ transplants has also forced us to look at how we define death, and to change our definition of death from a traditional one depending on the functions of the heart and lungs to a definition of brain death. Individuals and their families have had to ask the courts to intervene in the decision-making process concerning when a person is to be allowed to die.

Furthermore, we are confronting a new disease with no cure, AIDS. In the 1970s we did not know about AIDS. In the 1990s it is a leading cause of death. AIDS contradicts two myths: that we can contain death, and that death is only for the elderly.

As our attitudes toward death and dying change, death should become something we contemplate rather than a problem we must solve. Ultimately, "discussions of death must be discussions about life." The question must not be "How should we order our dying?"; but "How should we order our living?" (Steinfels, Note 5).

REFERENCE NOTES

1. Aries, P. *Western attitudes toward death*. Baltimore: Johns Hopkins University Press, 1974 and *The hour of our death*. New York: Vintage Books, 1982.
2. Samuel Pepys, as quoted in Thomlinson, R. *Population dynamics*. New York: Random House, 1966, p. 84.
3. Toynbee, A. Changing attitudes toward death in the modern western world. In A. Toynbee, A. K. Man, N. Smart, et al. (eds.) *Man's concern with death*. New York: McGraw-Hill, 1968, p. 131.
4. Rosenblatt, P. *Bitter, bitter tears*. Minneapolis: University of Minnesota Press, 1983, p. 66.
5. Steinfels, P. "Introduction." In P. Steinfels and R. Veatch (eds.) *Death inside out*. New York: Harper and Row, 1975, pp. 3–4.

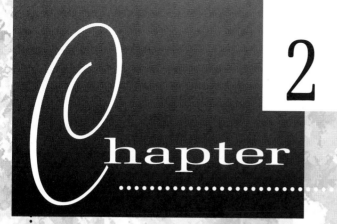

Chapter 2

Death and the Process of Dying

Today more than ever, urgent social issues such as euthanasia, AIDS, and capital punishment, and behaviors such as alcohol and drug abuse and certain acts of violence affect our perception of death. Throughout history, numerous interpretations and perceptions of death have existed in various cultures. The psychiatrist Carl Jung, for example, saw life and death as part of a continuing process, directed toward a goal that Jung called a state of rest. Similarly the expression often used when someone dies, "she passed . . . ," suggest a perception of death as a process in which one moves from this life to another.

The next life may be seen as a continuation of the familiar life on earth, it may assume more spiritual aspects, or it may be one of tribulation and pain. Hindus, Buddhists, and members of certain other religions that incorporate a belief in reincarnation view the embodied self as passing through childhood, youth, and old age; at death we leave that body and assume another one. In this view death is a chance for rebirth, or a transition between one form of life and another. On the other hand, for the Xhosa people of South Africa, death represents a transition from the world of flesh to the world of the departed, or the ancestral spirits. Others perceive death simply as a leveler, for despite power, money, or fame, each person will eventually die.

In the United States, our perceptions of death are exemplified in the elaborate funerals we arrange. These ceremonies serve as a last statement to society about the quality of a person's life, and to show the esteem felt by the survivors for the dead person. At a funeral, the survivors participate in a social rite of passage that validates their status in the community as well as the status of the deceased.

If, then, death is viewed as a part of the process of life as well as a separate event, we should examine the influence of human growth and development on our perceptions of death.

DEVELOPMENTAL INFLUENCES ON PERCEPTIONS OF DEATH

Within the psychosocial context of American culture, there are age-related characteristics that color and shape the meaning of death and dying for each person. For the child under the age of 3, illness and death are sources of separation anxiety. The very young child is concerned with physical comfort and knowing that his or her parent or consistent caregiver is available. Children at this age do not understand why a parent has left them unprotected and they may feel angry and abandoned. Preschoolers, age 3 to 5, often experience feelings of shame and mutilation of their bodies if they become ill. Illness may be viewed as a punishment and an obstruction to their growing sense of independence. Among school-age children 6 to 10, major concerns focus on an increased sense of competency and mastery. Their own illness may challenge this development. In addition, the school-age child may feel responsible for the illness or death of parents/siblings, attributing it to their own bad thoughts or actions. It is essential, therefore, that parents and caregivers of children in these three age groups provide a constancy of caring to lessen the fears of abandonment. Children should be given every opportunity to gain mastery over their situation.

The next developmental stage, adolescence, is a time of intense emotional and intellectual preoccupation. The adolescent is dealing with issues of consolidation of ego identity, emotional separation from the family, and a greater investment in the peer group. Adolescents can be extremely sensitive about their physical appearance: their image is very important, both to themselves and for how they feel others view them. Some psychologists assert that the adolescent does not have a sense of longevity and therefore develops a romantic notion of death. Adolescents are less concerned with the quantity of life than its quality, seeking affirmation of their worthiness and sense of self.

Hospitalization and illness therefore have an impact on adolescents' growing sense of self. Teenagers involved in the process of separation from parental authority now find themselves in a situation where all decisions concerning their body are left to their parents. Health care staff, if sensitive enough, may discuss procedures and the like with them, but parents are the ones who sign the consent forms. If the adolescent objects to a decision, this objection is often met with, "You're not old enough to decide." Furthermore, the disease or the treatment may involve loss of hair, weight, and energy. It is important, therefore, that adolescents' caregivers continue to affirm and confirm that the adolescent is a unique and real human being.

For the young adult, independent life is just beginning; developmental tasks in this period include establishing a work identity and intimacy with a loved partner, including perhaps marriage and having children. Facing death at this stage of the life cycle is overwhelmingly frustrating and disappointing. The young adult feels cheated and often speaks about how "unfair" life can be. Some individuals will cope with death by expressing rage at the world or by turning their rage inward and becoming depressed.

In one instance, a 22-year-old woman with bone cancer became increasingly depressed and refused to see visitors. When asked to share her feelings, she screamed, "Talking isn't going to help. Unless you can give me back the use of my legs so I can get on with my life, you're useless to me." In addition, if the individual has a spouse or life partner, or children, he or she may worry about who will care for these people.

The middle years of life have a deeper, interpersonal tone. This is a time of meaningful ongoing relationships, attainment of work goals, and expansion of the self. Energy is directed to establishing and guiding the next generation. It is also a time when many middle-aged people experience a parental death. Then that person is faced with the double task of incorporating a major loss and facing personal mortality. Shifting economic and employment trends may contribute to the stress and feelings of loss during this developmental age. In a popular book on middle age, the author commented that "the greatest burden we carry into middle age is the burden of our masks. To some degree each of us is an island. We devote enormous amounts of time and energy to keeping up appearances and maintaining a good front while each of us weeps in the privacy of our own souls" (Leshan, Note 1).

People facing death during this phase of life must reconcile themselves to losing the opportunity to enjoy family and life successes, as well as new horizons of growth, and to missing the experience of guiding the next generation. A 50-year-old man hospitalized with leukemia, for example, spoke about his sadness at having a terminal illness. He realized he probably would not see his 15-year-old son finish high school, and that he would not know his "potential grandchildren." He desperately hoped that he would have a year or so of retirement, because since he was a child he had always had to work. Now that he had achieved some financial stability, he wanted to experience what it would be like not to be "on the job 12 hours a day, six days a week. I couldn't allow myself the time then that I really deserved—I always promised myself 'later.'"

The older person faces multiple contradictions. This is the time when one is supposed to sit back and take life easy, but it is often a period of multiple losses: the loss of a spouse, peers, one's health, and work. It is what has been called "a time of bereavement overload." This is a period when the individual thinks about death in practical terms. The elderly person may fear that he or she will become burdensome, and may welcome death as an escape from an otherwise unbearable situation, as in the case of a recently widowed 89-year-old woman who was admitted to the hospital because of increasing weakness and periods of dizziness. Prior to her hospitalization, she had lived with her daughter, son-in-law, and five grandchildren. She very much wanted to return there, but said: "I know I can't go back. I feel like such a burden. None of this makes sense anymore. I've outlived my usefulness. Why doesn't God just take me?" However, although some older people may welcome death, the thought may also be accompanied by fear and anxiety.

FEAR OF DEATH AND DYING, AND DEATH ANXIETY

The literature about death and dying frequently refers to the fear of death and to death anxiety. The word *fear* ordinarily means that one is afraid of a specific thing or person, while anxiety, on the other hand, conjures up vague, uneasy feelings. Death is specific enough to fear yet sufficiently vague to cause anxiety. There are many unknowns associated with death that create anxiety: the uncertainty of how, when, and where death will come; of what will happen to survivors; of what it means to cease to exist.

Another distinction should be made between fear of death and fear of dying. Research indicates that some people may fear dying more than they fear death, for dying connotes weakness, pain, dependency, loss of control, change in body image, and loss of contact with others. To express a fear of dying may also be a defense against an actual fear of death, whose finality may be intensely frightening.

Helping people express their actual fears may be useful. Depending on the individual's fear, different avenues can be opened for possible relief. One hypothesis is that by "practicing death," that is, by reflecting on mortality, one may overcome a fear of it. Talking about death does not so much inform us about death as it reminds us about it little by little, again and again, and these reminders allow us to fit the event of death into our lives. For example, in a report on one discussion group in which the participants talked about their own deaths, results of a questionnaire completed three months after the discussions indicated that more than half of the participants felt that their fear of death and dying was reduced.

Study after study has shown that most people, even those who are at risk for higher mortality rates, *say* that they do not fear death. One study indicated that, in terms of race and sex differences, whites and men were statistically more likely to mention fear of death, while African-American women expressed the least fear of death. Thus, while people in general may have some death anxiety, the commonly held assumption that Americans have excessive fear or anxiety regarding death appears not to be true.

However, what people say on a questionnaire and what they actually feel and do may be very different.

The fear of extinction, annihilation, obliteration, or ceasing to be comprises the basic fear of death for most people (Kastenbaum and Aisenberg, Note 2). Ceasing to be is a difficult concept. Fear of the unknown can also be part of the fear of death and dying. What happens after death is simply not known; there is no TV camera crew to tape this event. Death evokes a feeling of ultimate powerlessness, since for most people, the time and cause of death are unpredictable.

Adding to this feeling of powerlessness is society's emphasis on independence and the control of one's own destiny. Loss of consciousness is frightening, because this symbolizes loss of self-mastery. Dying may also bring with it loss of control of bodily functions, such as urination and defecation, and people may fear disrespect and humiliation in needing assistance with such functions. Some research studies suggest that more specific planning for, and thus more control over, the dying process can lower death anxiety and avoid stressful crisis-oriented decisions at a very sad and painful time.

Another reason for fearing death may be that in death, it is no longer possible to achieve. To some, death represents the end of opportunities to affirm one's self by means of committed actions. Part of the source of this fear may lie within America's goal-oriented culture and in the fact for some people, self-esteem is related to what they produce, what projects they complete, and how much money they make. Thus, one psychiatrist has hypothesized that when individuals feel they have completed their life's work, they are ready to die.

Fear of death may also be related to a dread of isolation or separation, the deprivation of one of our most basic human needs, intimacy with other human beings. Death, the ultimate separation, may be seen as total isolation and aloneness, a state of being that is intolerable to most people. In Tolstoy's *The Death of Ivan Ilyich*, readers can sense the anguish in Ivan's fear of the unknown and separation when he says: "Yes, life was there and now it is going, going and I cannot stop it. Yes. Why deceive myself? Isn't it obvious to everyone but me that I'm dying, and that it's only a question of weeks, days, . . . it may happen this moment. There was light and now there is darkness. I was here and now I'm going there! Where?" (Tolstoy, Note 3).

Finally, people may fear death in terms of what will become of their dependents—their children, their spouse, their elderly parents. Nevertheless they are often reluctant to make out a will for the distribution of their material accumulations. Writing a will forces individuals to take an additional step in contemplating their own death, a step that many people resist to avoid weighing the possibility of dying. When people enter the medical care system as patients, however, caregivers can and do assess their potential for dying at a particular time.

DYING AS A PROCESS

Patients entering a medical care institution set into motion a number of immediate responses on the part of professional caregivers. Staff must determine a diagnosis for the patient that in turn helps to establish what the projected course of illness will be; what, where, and when interventions can occur; and what the prognosis will be. Once a physician arrives at a diagnosis of a terminal illness for a patient, the patient enters a "dying trajectory," a curve along which the terminal illness moves.

There are various types of dying trajectories. In the trajectory for accidents, for example, when a person is in an immediately life-threatening situation, the time frame for resolving dying issues is quite clear. In the trajectory typical of chronic fatal illness, however, death will occur at an unknown time. In a third type of trajectory, as when a person requires radical surgery and will need to go through that crisis to obtain a prognosis, the certainty of death is unknown. And in illnesses due to genetic diseases, HIV infection, or multiple sclerosis, for example, the time and certainty of death is unclear, and people must live with the ambiguity associated with these diagnoses. Patients themselves may also influence their dying trajectories. In one case where medical personnel had little hope for a patient's recovery from a severe illness, the patient's own prescription for healing, which included experiencing humor, facilitated his ultimate recovery.

Along the dying trajectory, certain junctures or stages are passed: the patient is defined as dying; staff and family prepare for the patient's death; it is decided that nothing more can be done; the final descent occurs leading to the last hours and the death watch; and finally the death itself occurs. Caregivers must determine the critical junctures with care, so they will feel that they have done the most that was possible for the patient.

Perceptions of the dying process may be different for the caregiver and the patient. In her book *On Death and Dying*, Kübler-Ross divided the patient's perception of the process of dying into five phases (Kübler-Ross, Note 4).

In the first stage, denial and isolation, Kübler-Ross found that once patients were informed that they were dying, they could not believe the prognosis was true. This may be a healthy way of dealing with this painful information. Denial can function as a buffer after the unexpected news, and it allows people to collect themselves and mobilize other defenses. After learning of his diagnosis of inoperable cancer, for instance, one patient stated: "I'm relieved that surgery isn't necessary—now I can take my vacation and return to work. Surgery would have interfered with my plans."

Denial then gives way to feelings of rage, resentment, and envy. In this second stage of anger, patients ask themselves the question, Why me? Anger may also be projected toward the people around them. For example, one 25-year-old patient dying of cancer smashed an IV bottle because a nurse had not responded to her call for help quickly enough.

In the third stage, bargaining, there is an attempt to postpone death. People may bargain with God to gain more time. Usually family events or projects are mentioned. "I've asked God to let me live until my daughter takes her first step." "God knows I have a good book in me. I'm sure this chemotherapy will give me enough time to finish it."

Depression is the fourth stage. When terminally ill patients can no longer deny that they are dying, often because of increasingly severe signs and symptoms of disease, such as pain and weight loss, the anger and rage are replaced by feelings of depression and great loss. This is a phase of anticipatory grief that one may experience in order to prepare for death.

Finally, if patients have had enough time and have been able to experience the previous four phases, they may well reach a stage of acceptance of their dying. Feelings of anger, depression, and loss are no longer powerful but become distant, with the patient's focus on dying. Patients in this phase may turn inward with their thoughts and feelings, and their circle of interests may diminish. Families may need more help, support, and understanding than the patients at this time.

Kübler-Ross's work on these five stages has become an accepted model for the care of the dying, although caregivers should not view the stages as normative. Rather, they may be used as a descriptive tool to understand the dying process. In addition, thanatologists suggest that the five stages do not always progress in a linear fashion. Not all patients experience all five stages, and some patients may alternate between acceptance and denial, with these and other stages not being mutually exclusive. Other thanatologists have stated, too, that these five stages may not be applicable to the vast majority of people who die in old age. For while death of a middle-aged person may be untimely, the death of an older person may be expected and accepted. Elderly people may experience a gradual decrease in physical vitality over a period of time. They may make accommodations to such changes and still remain active in their lives.

Whatever the professionals' theory about the stages of dying, perhaps one general conclusion to draw is that dying may evoke a number of emotions, such as anger, sadness, depression, and relief, and that these emotions do not occur in any specific order. People who are dying, however, must cope not only with their own emotions but also with societal responses to death and dying.

STIGMA AND THE DYING PERSON

A stigma may be attached to the dying person because that person represents what people fear about their own death; he or she shatters people's immortal image of themselves and the plans they have made for the future. The dying patient is also a deviant in the medical subculture, because death threatens the image of the physician as healer and the goal of curing patients in acute-care hospital settings. When a person is labeled as a deviant, that individual is stigmatized. One study of attitudes toward the terminally ill, for example, found the existence of more negative attitudes toward the dying than are generally found expressed toward the ill or the healthy. Values and attitudes that result in the practice of isolating people who are dying, and of not speaking openly about dying, support the idea of death as a stigma and the feeling that certain diseases are more feared than others. The stigma of death can thus also be transferred to a specific disease entity.

Many people believe that the diagnosis of cancer is synonymous with death, that the word *cancer* is so powerful that a patient's knowledge of this diagnosis can actually hasten death. Relatives and friends may request that a patient not be told of this diagnosis because "it will kill her," as if the knowledge and not the disease would be the cause of death. Once patients are told of a diagnosis of cancer, they must cope not only with personal fears but with those of relatives, friends, health care professionals, and society at large. These fears manifest themselves in a variety of ways, and cancer patients may be confronted with isolation from friends ("I don't know what to say"), loss of employment ("How can a dying person work?"), and neglect or indifference from the medical staff ("There's nothing more to do"). This diagnosis may so alter the image of individuals, both to themselves and others, that they become "different."

On the other hand, the cardiac patient faces none of these dilemmas. It would seem foolish not to inform a patient of a cardiac condition. Family and friends do not worry about what to say to cardiac patients about their disease. To the contrary, what led to the heart attack, courses of treatment, and anticipated outcomes are frequent topics of conversation in visits with these patients. Employers often encourage employees with heart disease "to take it easy" and arrange for less stressful assignments on their return to work. Yet cardiovascular diseases claimed 982,574 lives in 1988 while cancer claimed 488,240 lives (American Heart Association, Note 5). Recent figures provided by the American Cancer Society indicate that four of ten patients who get cancer in 1991 will be alive five years after diagnosis. Statistics therefore would seem to support our being less cancer phobic and more cardiac phobic. Why is this not so?

Susan Sontag, in her widely read book *Illness as a Metaphor*, suggests that the labels, notions, and myths about an illness create a metaphor that transforms the illness and gives it a special meaning. She postulates that cancer lends itself to a metaphor because it is "intractable and capricious—it is a disease not understood—in an era in which medicine's central premise is that all diseases can be cured" (Sontag, Note 6). Or, as another author describes cancer, "It is a crab. . . . It claws at us, it hides in the sands of our flesh; like a crab it ignores straight walking, progressing sideways both in its refusal to behave in an honest, purposeful manner and in its need to invade neighboring tissues" (Richards, Note 7).

The metaphor will continue until the cause and cure of cancer are found. Fear of the unknown is universal, and it takes on special meaning for cancer patients. They have the image of something unknown growing in their body. They search for a meaning; since the disease appears so irrational, it evokes irrational responses. Patients may even view the disease as punishment and experience feelings of guilt, shame, and disgust.

Also part of the unknown etiology is a fear of contagion. Although many consider Americans to be sophisticated in these matters, there are still people who worry that being around a cancer patient may be dangerous. One relative, a successful, prominent lawyer, spoke about his feelings regarding his mother: "I know this sounds foolish, but I found myself not wanting to touch her. I became worried. We really didn't know the cause of cancer. My solution was to hire someone to care for her."

A cancer patient also faces a rigorous treatment regime that may temporarily or permanently affect the body image. Surgery often results in physical disfigurement. Patients with colostomies worry about offensive odors and having "accidents." Patients who have had mastectomies are reassured that a breast prosthesis or implant will be so lifelike that it will escape detection by the outside world, but such reassurances are a double-edged sword, for the implicit message is that there is something to hide. Cancer patients may also fear that they are no longer sexually attractive. And as Sontag notes, we assign a hierarchy to our organs, and cancer frequently occurs in parts of the body that we are embarrassed to acknowledge—for example, the colon, bladder, rectum, breast, prostate gland.

Unlike cancer patients, cardiac patients know the etiology of their disease. It is often site specific and not the result of "cellular derangement." They can experience more control over the progress and treatment of their disease. A malfunctioning heart may be "fixed" by medication, surgery, diet, and modification of life-style. Cardiac patients rarely are worried that they are no longer sexually attractive; their anxiety is related to the idea that sexual activity may precipitate another attack.

Also, the type of death associated with each of these diseases is very different. Cancer is associated with prolonged illness, increasing debilitation and dependency, unrelieved pain, and the knowledge that one is dying. Cardiac death suggests a fast, relatively painless death that comes without warning. The stigma attached to dying, then, may relate not only to fear of death, social attitudes and values, and a specific disease, but also to the actual process of dying.

Probably in no other situation do all these factors gather together so clearly as in the stigma attached to AIDS and HIV infection. AIDS, as opposed to cancer and cardiac disease, is a communicable, sexually transmitted disease associated with terminal illness. In addition, the greatest impact of this disease so far has been on already socially stigmatized groups including gay and bisexual men and intravenous (IV) drug users. The indigent, African-Americans, and Latinos are also disproportionately affected. And the increasing number of women with AIDS and HIV have remained a forgotten group in the epidemic. The public views these women as transmitters of the disease to their children and male sexual partners, rather than as people with AIDS who are themselves frequently victims of transmission from the men in their lives. Since AIDS has predominantly affected men, it has been identified by signs and symptoms characteristic of male responses. The signs and symptoms of the disease in women have not been clearly delineated. Women with AIDS may find physicians not especially responsive to their illness, and the disease may be in a fairly advanced stage before it is even diagnosed.

Up until the past few years, AIDS was synonymous with death, evoking fear of death even among health care providers. That association is now not always made. Many people with AIDS and HIV have begun to resist death as an inevitable outcome. This has been facilitated by the advent of new treatment and medication regimens that support living with the disease as a chronic illness for longer periods of time. In addition, people with AIDS and HIV may turn to complementary therapies, such as acupuncture, meditation, massage, guided imagery, and spiritual healing.

The more that people can identify with persons who have AIDS and HIV, the less they will fear them. Research shows that social interaction decreases fear of contagion, probably because it increases sensitivity to the concerns of those infected, thus removing the cultural associations of disgrace. It is important, then, to get to know persons with AIDS and HIV, to become aware of their values, hopes, and changing dreams for their lives in relation to this disease, and to recognize the shared humanity in all of our experiences. To do this, the issue of talking with people about their terminal illness and their dying must be considered.

TALKING WITH PEOPLE ABOUT THEIR DYING

Knowing when and how to talk with dying patients and their families about death-related issues continues to be an area of concern for many health care providers. The reasons for such concern are multiple and may include personal feelings of inadequacy, avoidance of potentially distressing situations, peer pressure against open talk, and prohibitions by physicians or family against conversation with the patient concerning his or her diagnosis and prognosis. The judgment, however, about what a dying person should be told is very much connected to deeply rooted social, cultural, and psychological patterns.

Physicians have traditionally been the professionals to disclose a diagnosis of terminal illness. Studies done 30 to 40 years ago about physician disclosure indicate that they were reluctant to tell patients about a serious or terminal prognosis. In contrast, studies done in the 1970s and 1980s show that a large majority of physicians apparently do inform patients of their dying status. Younger physicians in particular are more likely to tell a dying patient about his or her terminal prognosis.

Changes in beliefs and values in the underlying social structure, and major restructuring of the health care delivery system, may be seen as influencing this trend toward disclosure. For example, the traditional one-to-one relationship between patient and physician in which the physician is viewed as a benign but authoritarian figure and the patient's role is one of passive recipient has changed. Physicians are more willing now to recognize the principles of patient autonomy and self-determination. And as American society becomes more consumer oriented, and as health care is seen more in terms of disease prevention and self-care, people are becoming more protective of their rights to self-determination.

This right to self-determination has become increasingly evident as technology allows patients to survive on life-support machines. People are now concerned about their right to die and the legal recognition of living wills. The current social value of informed consent requires disclosure of the prognosis and effects of nontreatment so that the patient can make a knowledgeable decision for treatment, and this value is reflected legally as well. Congress has passed legislation requiring all Medicare and Medicaid providers to inform patients, on admission, of their right to refuse treatment. This law was intended to remind people to make their wishes known by drawing up a living will or by granting a durable power of attorney. Many states have enacted do-not-resuscitate laws, which require physicians to discuss with hospital patients their wishes regarding the use of resuscitation if they should experience a life-threatening episode. As this trend continues patients will increasingly expect the physician and other caregivers to act as technical experts and advisers and to invite and include patient participation in treatment plans.

These new roles for patients and caregivers are developing within the context of a major restructuring of the health care delivery system in the United States. As it is now, however, patients receive treatment within a huge health care bureaucracy involving inpatient, outpatient, and home care, with numerous professionals providing the care for one person. Disclosure of prognosis to the patient becomes a much more critical issue, as the danger of miscommunication among staff and between staff and patient can easily occur, given the number of people involved. The patient is at risk for confusion and distress if mixed messages are received from caregivers. It is therefore important for caregivers to communicate with other members of the health team as to what patients have been told about their diagnosis and prognosis. A team assessment of the patient's need to know about a diagnosis of a terminal illness is helpful. However, nurses, physicians, and social workers are expected by patients and society to use judgment and discretion in the disclosure of information.

Patients will vary in their need to be aware that they are dying and in their ability to cope with that knowledge. It is important to assess very carefully the patients' and families' understanding of the disease involved, their ways of dealing with stress and crises in the past as well as the present, their cultural orientation to death and grieving, and their support systems. In China, for example, aggressive treatment is maintained right to the moment of death, and while the family is informed if the patient's disease is terminal, it seems that the patient is not. In Japan, too, the vast majority of physicians still avoid informing a patient of a malignant illness (Taka-hashi, Note 8). This is not only related to physicians' fears but also to the Japanese culture's emphasis on interdependence. To declare that a patient has a malignant illness may mean not only that the person is dying but also that important relationships of interdependence with other people are destroyed.

There seem to be no set rules about what and how much patients should be told about the diagnosis of their terminal illness. Listening to patients talk about their illness and their knowledge of the outcome can reveal a great deal. If patients say they feel upset, they can be encouraged to talk about that feeling; if they make such statements as, "Well, I don't think I'll need this medicine much longer," they need to be encouraged to clarify that. If caregivers provide careful listening and attentive responses, there will be little for them to actually "tell."

It is also important for caregivers to provide people with information at the pace at which they desire it. People who are dying do not allow them-selves to hear more than they are ready to accept at a given moment. Patients deserve a thorough assessment of their needs and of their abilities to cope with the knowledge of their dying.

COPING WITH DEATH AND DYING

How a person copes with her or his own dying differs with each individ-ual. Coping strategies utilized with a life-threatening illness may differ from those strategies used to deal with non-life-threatening situations such as the loss of a job. In a study conducted with terminally ill patients about their expectations of nurses, it emerged that five factors characterize the kind of assistance individuals may need to cope with dying (Arblaster et al., Note 9). The first three, normalcy, empowerment, and autonomy, focus on individual needs; the remaining two factors, support and partnership, focus primarily on family needs.

For many people, coping with dying involves an emphasis on "keeping things normal." Support and care are needed to maintain the status quo as much as possible within the individual's life and within the family unit. One person said, for example, "I feel like people are seeing me differ-ently—I have another dimension now. I don't feel differently towards them. They feel like I'm having a mystical experience. With my family, I plan on normalcy—on the living—not the dying."

Dying persons, of course, want freedom from pain, but they also express the desire to be able to think clearly, to be able to love, and to be loved in return. Dying persons also have plans for the future. Important in the factor of empowerment are the concepts of dying persons and caregivers sharing equally in decision making and of people wanting to control their lives. Therefore the dying person is not perceived as subordinate to caregivers, but as a person able to choose a course of treatment with which she or he feels comfortable. Identification of each person's agenda with regard to dying is vital. Caregivers can empower a patient by asking, for example, "What would you still like to do?" Empowerment enhances the person's decision-making abilities.

Autonomy is related to empowerment and is equally important. People are encouraged to participate in their own care to the extent that they desire. If dying people are physically unable to participate in their care, they nevertheless may be able to participate in decision making. A person may decide, for example, to deal with pain quite differently at its inception than several months later. Those who are dying want to be as independent as possible for as long as possible. Hospital staff need to think in terms of "working with" rather "doing to" the patients, and open and honest communication is an important component here.

Partnership and support, like the other factors in this coping framework, must be assessed in terms of the individual and his or her family situation—patient autonomy, family involvement, issues of family dynamics, and coping mechanisms. The focus of care may vary; some families may not be able to be involved, and some dying people may not want their families involved.

Recognizing people's individual ways of experiencing life and death is an important beginning in assisting them in coping with their dying. People may be able to experience comfortable dying and dying with dignity if they can be helped to identify their agenda for their remaining life, and helped to carry it out. Supporting the integrity of dying people in this way may provide them with the opportunity to bring closure to their life.

REFERENCE NOTES

1. Leshan, E. *The wonderful crisis of middle age.* New York: D. McKay, 1973.
2. Kastenbaum, R., & Aisenberg, R. *The psychology of death.* New York: Springer, 1972.

3. Tolstoy, L. *The death of Ivan Ilyich and other stories.* New York: New American Library, 1960, 129–130.
4. Kübler-Ross, E. *On death and dying.* New York: Macmillan, 1969.
5. American Heart Association. *1991 heart and stroke facts.* National Center, Dallas, Texas: American Heart Association, 1991.
6. Sontag, S. *Illness as metaphor.* New York: Vintage Books, 1979.
7. Richards, V. *Cancer: The wayward cell.* Berkeley: University of California Press, 1972.
8. Takahashi, Y. Informing a patient of malignant illness: Commentary from a cross-cultural perspective. *Death studies*, 1990, *14* (1), 83–91.
9. Arblaster, G., Brooks, D., Hudson, R., & Petty, M. Terminally ill patients' expectations of nurses. *Australian Journal of Advanced Nursing*, 1990, *7* (3), 34–43.

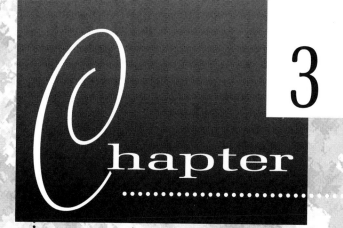

Chapter 3

The Helping Professions and the Terminally Ill

The challenges of caring for people who are terminally ill can be immense, the rewards fulfilling and worthwhile. However, the experience can evoke a spectrum of human emotions ranging from confusion, grief, helplessness, fear, and anger to intimacy, love, and pity. The caregiver may want the person to live or to die; he or she may feel committed and entrapped, protective and alienated, all at the same time. Providing care can offer caregivers new perspectives on their own lives and what it means to be human. But the challenges involved in caring for people who are terminally ill may also result in exhaustion, burnout, and even career changes for caregivers.

NURSES

Nurses are the professional caregivers who are in the most continuous contact with dying patients—in institutions and in the home—and who provide them with the most direct care. Nurses face their own fears, anxieties, and concerns about death each time they help a patient to die in dignity and peace.

In the 1960s nurse educators began to address the issue of adding death education to the nursing curriculum. Yet, while many nursing schools today have integrated concepts and issues concerning death and dying into their courses, the amount of time devoted to the subject is small, and there are few required courses in death education. Furthermore, most schools of nursing do not systematically assign students to dying patients. If students do not integrate their learning in clinical practice, they are not receiving the maximum benefit from their instruction.

Research suggests that specific death education courses reduce nursing students' death anxiety and improve attitudes toward patient care. Research also suggests that nurses with high and moderate exposure to dying patients were found to be significantly more comfortable with them than were nurses with low exposure. Through specific education in death and dying, nurses may develop the self-awareness that forms a significant basis of their interactions with terminally ill patients.

All nurses are familiar with assessment, the first step of the nursing process used to collaborate with patients in initiating, planning, and evaluating their nursing care. In caring for dying patients, nurses need to assess their own feelings and responses about death, as well as those of their patients. Otherwise, nurses are in danger of imposing their own beliefs and judgments about death on their patients, assuming an authoritarian role rather than the advocacy role that is a function of nursing. This difference becomes especially important when nurses are faced with moral dilemmas in the care of dying people, such as the continuation of life-support systems. It is vital that nurses understand death at the philosophical, the clinical, and the personal level so that they will be equipped to make complex ethical decisions.

Values clarification may be needed as part of developing nurses' self-awareness, because often dying patients have life-styles different than those of caregivers. Nurses care for patients who are dying from AIDS, drug overdoses, chronic and acute illnesses, accidents, gunshot and stab wounds. Obtaining some clarity about one's own personal values and one's feelings toward patients is necessary for an understanding of the professional responses that are required in providing care.

As nurses face conflicts of both personal and professional identity in caring for dying patients, personal death anxieties may surface. Discussing death with a patient can evoke fear, sadness, and anger about one's own mortality and powerlessness. These are uncomfortable and disturbing feelings in a society and a profession in which keeping one's emotions in control is emphasized. Also, in our highly technological and scientific society, death may represent both personal and professional failure, since nurses are educated to anticipate any untoward events that may place patients at risk and to plan appropriate interventions to prevent them.

Nurses and the Dying Patient

People who are dying may become increasingly dependent on nurses for assistance in activities of daily living such as personal hygiene, nutrition and elimination, and exercise. How nurses provide this assistance is critically important for the patient not only physiologically but also psychologically, because nursing care can convey basic respect or disrespect for the patient as a human being.

Conveyance of respect begins as nurses collaborate with patients in planning their nursing care. Even if patients are totally dependent on the nursing staff, they may still be able to take part in decisions such as when they will have a bath, a dressing change, pain medication, or whether or not they want visitors that day. One nurse asks her patients each morning, "What are your plans for today?" She then works with each patient to decide how to schedule activities, rest, treatments, and visitors throughout the day.

The actual touching involved in providing physical care may also be critical. The concept of "therapeutic touch," or laying hands on or close to the body of an ill person for the purpose of helping or healing, is useful to keep in mind. A child in pain in a hospital once said to a nurse, "Touch me where it hurts." Adults in American culture may find it difficult to ask to be held or touched. It is far easier and acceptable to ask for medication. In addition, those who are dying, besides often experiencing pain, may feel unclean or repulsive, or that there is an unpleasant odor about them that will keep people away. People with AIDS may feel that others do not want to touch them because of fear of contagion. Therefore, how nurses touch patients when providing nursing care can convey acceptance, respect, and caring.

The day-to-day physical care and the emotional and psychological support that dying patients require continually taps into nurses' personal resources and energy levels. Nurses do not have the mobility on hospital units that physicians and social workers do, to come and go throughout the day, evening, or night; nurses remain on the unit with the patients. Although this can be problematic at times in terms of nurses' own need to obtain some distance from the situation even for a short time, it also provides them with a unique experience—being present when patients need a moment to share with someone. One patient, dying in a hospital, asked a night nurse to stop and hold his hand for a few minutes when she made her rounds, even if he was asleep. He simply said, "I don't want to be alone."

Nurses coordinate the treatment and decisions made by the various people involved in caring for the dying person. Providing comfort to dying patients involves collaboration with the patients in deciding on their plan of care, facilitating their decisions about day-to-day living, encouraging open communication between them and those close to them, and sustaining them in the maintenance of their dignity, self-worth, and self-respect throughout their dying.

One study of nurses caring for the terminally ill on a coronary care unit found that nurses did not report severe coping difficulties associated with their care of dying patients. Rather, their most severe difficulties were those related to telling relatives about a patient's death. Organizational structures that eased coping responses included a high staff-patient ratio, low staff turnover, supportive relationships among staff, and a policy of open and honest communication about prognosis.

When nurses experience feelings of powerlessness or personal and professional failure when caring for dying patients, they may use negative coping strategies, such as avoidance, to deal with their conflicts and anxieties. Nurses may avoid interacting with patients by evading conversation, by briskness and efficiency in providing physical care, by speaking only when spoken to by the patient, and by restricting conversation to topics that are comfortable for the nurse. One nurse realized that she was avoiding her dying patients by telling herself, "I'm too busy," "Someone else can profit more from my care," "He needs the rest," or "She prefers to be alone." When she saw what she was doing, this nurse discovered that she could indeed schedule 20 to 30 minutes of each working day to be with a dying patient. Other defense mechanisms used by staff members to distance themselves from terminally ill patients may include denial and psychiatric labeling, by assigning different nurses to dying patients each day, and by doing routine work before spending time talking with patients.

However, given the nursing care needs of acutely ill patients, nursing staff must frequently triage their patients. A priority assessment must be made as to which patients require professional nursing care. If there is a shortage of registered professional nurses, nursing staff may have to delegate care of terminally ill patients to nurses' aides or "float" nurses (those assigned to that unit for just one day) because of the acute care needs of other patients.

Individual characteristics, such as a nurse's age, nursing experience, personal experiences with dying people, and death anxiety, may contribute to the degree and quality of patient interaction, as may organizational structures of specialty units, the number of nurses on staff, and interdisciplinary staff relationships. The interaction of these factors also influences nurses' responses to and behavior toward dying patients' families.

Nurses and the Family Unit

The concept of the patient and patient's family as being the unit of care is a significant one in working with dying patients. Thinking of the whole family as a unit can promote an understanding of how the health or illness of one member influences the well-being of other members and affects the functioning of the total family group. Spouses of patients who are critically ill may experience intense feelings of impending loss. Hospitalization of the patient may enhance these feelings, as the spouse experiences interruption in daily routines including sleep and meal patterns, forced autonomy, drastic role reversals, possible loss of financial support, and interruption of an interpersonal reward system. If the patient has been chronically ill, the family's physical and emotional resources may already be depleted, with little reserve left to cope with impending death. Nurses who use the framework of the patient and family as the unit of care focus on collaborating with all family members, including the patient, in assessing and planning the care that is needed by that unit.

In one survey of family caregivers in a home-based hospice program, family members reported the following caregiving needs: communication with professionals, assistance with patient care, legal matters, religious concerns, and household tasks. Another study found that the social support requirements of families of terminal cancer patients also included provision of information about patients' conditions or care from health care providers.

A third study, conducted to identify those nursing behaviors that provide the most support and comfort to loved ones of the terminally ill, hospitalized adult patient, showed that the four most desired behaviors were keeping the patient well groomed, allowing the patient to do as much for herself or himself as possible, giving the pain medication as often as possible (as indicated by physician's orders), and keeping the patient physically comfortable. The four least desired behaviors were encouraging the caregivers to cry, holding their hands, crying with them, and reminding them that the patient's suffering would be over soon. Similar studies have suggested that grieving family members may need nursing behaviors to be directed toward comforting, supporting, and easing the suffering of the dying patient rather than toward themselves. However, indications are that the most important family care need is the need for information: families want honest answers to their questions and specific information that might help them in caring for the patient.

In assessing and planning care with families of critically ill patients, nurses should consider the family's initial anxieties and informational concerns, the emotional support and interfamily contact required, and the personal needs of family members. Further, it is important to remember that family members may be in a crisis state of disequilibrium when first confronted with a loved one's diagnosis of terminal illness or the possibility of her or his impending death. Information needs to be presented clearly and simply, and perhaps repeated later. Family members can be encouraged to remain with the patient as much as is comfortably possible for themselves and the patient.

Open communication of both medical information and personal concerns is the key to emotional support. When patients and families sense permission within the hospital environment to acknowledge their emotional stress and pain, they are better able to release the tension that accompanies those feelings. Then they may feel less isolated, and less threatened by fears of losing control. Nurses and family members may explore together the coping strategies the family has used in past crises and whether it is helpful to continue these. New strategies may need to be developed. One hospice nurse, Kathleen MacInnis, writes to dying patients about making good-byes: "Get a confessor. Early on, find someone with whom you can talk 'dirty.' A friend, nurse, physician, or family member who will allow you to say words like 'dead, kick the bucket, croak, tumor, cancer.' All those things you—and your loved ones—are thinking but are too polite to say out loud. Say them. It won't hurt you and you'll feel better" (MacInnis, Note 1). This kind of open communication is not without its problems. At the time when a dying patient wants to talk about impending death, the listener may find the discussion unbearably painful. One husband responded to his wife's talking about her death by saying, "I feel I'm a victim of terminal candor."

Nurses can encourage family members and friends to keep in close contact with each other. They need to find out from relatives how they want to be notified if they are not there when the patient dies: it is difficult for a relative to be informed of death when alone, and every effort should be made to contact other family members and friends so that they can comfort each other at this time.

If the dying patient is in the hospital, families can be offered the opportunity to participate in the nursing care where circumstances permit. This may help them cope with feelings of helplessness and powerlessness. However, family members' varying degrees of desire and ability to participate need to be respected by the nursing staff. Patients should participate in these decisions, as both patients and family members may be apprehensive about the actual safety and technical aspects of providing care.

Family members assisting in the care of their relatives also need rest, relaxation, and some time of their own. They must receive adequate sleep and nutrition. A wife who is with her dying husband in the hospital every day may need a nurse to say to her: "We'll be here with him and call you if you're needed—why don't you go home and try to relax for a while?" Family caregivers of patients at home need to know about available alternatives when they need some respite from this care. They may also need support to help keep them from feeling like failures as caregivers if they do ask for help.

Emotional Issues

In the past, professional nurses were admonished: "Don't get emotionally involved with your patients"; "Don't get too close to the patients"; "You'll never make a good nurse if you can't control your feelings." Today, however, these admonitions have been put to rest. In cases where the traditional kinship network falters or family members disengage themselves from their dying relative, nurses and other caregivers may find themselves participating in the social and emotional support of their patients. They establish emotional bonds with their patients, and they are the ones, the health care team members, who may be there when the patient dies.

Painful feelings of loss and grief are just as normal for staff as they are for patients and family members. Just as patients often fear the process of dying—the loneliness, the isolation, the loss of dignity—more than death itself, so too nurses working with dying patients may fear the same isolation, and wonder who will be available to share their feelings of relief and sorrow, anger and acceptance, when patients die. Younger staff nurses may have a special need to discuss their feelings about a dying patient, particularly if the patient is another young adult of their same age. Older nurses who are trying to come to a realistic acceptance of their own mortality may also have a special need to talk about death and dying, especially if they are seeing themselves in each dying patient.

One workshop held for nursing staff working with chronically and terminally ill patients found that the most devastating issues in providing such nursing care were the following: anger and guilt, anxiety, lack of skills, overidentification, depression and sadness, and role confusion. Similarly, a professor discovered while teaching a seminar for nursing and medical students on the health professional as a survivor that the students did experience mourning and loss when patients died.

In some specialty areas such as pediatric intensive care units, where multiple deaths or other traumatic events often occur in rapid succession, there should be some opportunity for caregivers to process their own feelings before they are expected to provide demanding, potentially lifesaving care to other patients.

The nursing literature reflects nurses' needs for support and to grieve. Suggested tactics that can encourage nurses to care for themselves and, by doing so, to improve the quality of care to patients and families include the following:

- Exploring feelings about their own losses and identifying losses that they are still struggling to overcome
- Identifying resources that can help them deal with loss
- Reflecting about ideas of life after death
- Recognizing personal limitations
- Actively coping with a patient's death
- Reducing their own stress by practicing positive attitudes, exercising, and relaxing

Nurses can also provide support for each other through sharing their feelings about caring for terminally ill patients. Nurses working in an area where patient deaths are frequent may want to organize a monthly support group. Encouragement of informal peer support, such as giving each other "strokes," especially in times of stress, can be helpful at all levels of nursing. Educational experiences, such as conferences and workshops on death and dying designed to facilitate cognitive, affective, and personal learning, can be requested.

Consideration of unit and organizational system changes is important. Nurses caring for dying patients may need some daily period of time to examine their own feelings, to think about this experience. If a patient dies, they may need some time to prepare to care for the next patient. Formal systems of dealing with stress might involve time off for conferences, rotating different responsibilities on the unit, and mental health days. Nurses should also have a place where they can express powerful emotions in privacy, and hospitals might even offer special compensation for those involved with dying. As part of a bereavement and loss program, one intensive care unit set up a follow-up plan that allows staff to maintain contact with bereaved families in the months following the death.

Nurses, in collaboration with other health care professionals, patients, and families, will have to initiate these types of changes in our current disease-oriented, technological medical system if they wish to emphasize humanistic care for dying patients.

PHYSICIANS

The physicians' role is primarily as a healer of the sick. Physicians are supposed to have the knowledge to make correct medical judgments in moments of grave danger. The physician who shows indecision and worry will lose the confidence of his or her patients. Yet if a patient is dying, then the physician is not curing, nor can certainty be professed in treatment. The dying patient may come to represent the doctor's loss of power and control, especially as the medical care becomes more precarious.

One may discern four major issues in the goals of the physician vis-à-vis patient care: diagnosis, treatment, relief, and trust (Weisman, Note 2). Although the goal of diagnosis is the same for terminal and nonterminal patients, the other three goals take on different meanings in the care of the dying patient.

Treatment is usually considered to lead to curing. When the patient cannot be cured, however, the goal of the treatment changes: it may be to increase the length of the life of the patient; it may be to relieve the symptoms of the patient's illness; or it may be to satisfy the physician that he or she is doing everything possible. Clinical pathology conferences, or "death rounds," in which the medical staff involved discusses all the treatment options that might avoid death, may lead to cases of treatment for treatment's sake, for not only is the patient's life at stake, but the clinician's reputation and self-esteem are at risk as well.

One of the major difficulties for physicians in treating dying patients is that they confuse the dying role with the sick role (Noyes and Clancy, Note 3). A person in the sick role must want to get well, and must cooperate with the physician to achieve that end. The duty of dying persons is to desire to live as long as possible, and they must also cooperate with their caregivers. Sick people, for the limited time they are sick, are allowed to be dependent, whereas the dying are encouraged to be more independent and to care for themselves as much as possible. If the physician views the dying patient as if he or she is sick, both the physician and patient must then act as if the patient is improving. One result of this role confusion may be continual and active treatment for the patient.

From the dying patient's viewpoint, the doctor's primary goal must be one of relief: control and relief of pain. Yet medical personnel are not necessarily cognizant of the best methods of pain control for the terminally ill. Furthermore, while dying patients need to know that they can communicate their fears and their feelings, and that their questions will be answered honestly, physicians may find this particularly difficult, since they may see death as a failure on their part. The doctor's fantasy of being able to cure all patients is shattered. Safe conduct is another important goal from the dying patient's perspective. Such patients must trust that they will be taken care of with concern and dignity.

Because physicians have difficulties in achieving their goals with the terminally ill, they will generally respond in one of three ways to the dying patient: they may concentrate on the medical diagnosis and employ every technical skill to save the patient at all costs, they may practice avoidance and neglect, or they may exhibit detached but sympathetic support.

The first approach is exemplified by the physician who constantly is trying new treatments on his/her dying patient.

The second approach, avoidance and neglect, tends to develop as the "caring" aspect overshadows the "curing" aspect of treatment. Because there are few rewards for providing that care, the physician uses the rationalization of medical prioritizing to avoid the patient ("Nothing more can be done").

The physician who exhibits the third approach, detached-sympathetic support, will interact well with dying patients and be aware of their needs, but as one knowledgable writer has pointed out, these physicians are the mavericks, and there is little formal support of their nontechnical activities (Moller, Note 4).

Medical School Education

The process of socialization is the means by which persons acquire the knowledge and skills to perform in various roles. Medical school education is a primary component in the socialization of physicians. The format of medical education has basically remained the same since 1910. This features a clear separation between the basic and clinical science, a heavy use of lectures to large groups of students, and an emphasis on the teacher's role as an expert. The courses are poorly coordinated, and in the third and fourth years of school the student's main concern is his or her choice of residency.

The result of medical education is that first, there is a dehumanizing effect in the first two years of medical school (the preclinical years), since the student has no contact with patients while working on cadavers in pathology. Second, there is a compartmentalization effect implicit in the medical curriculum. During the preclinical years, the students study localized pathology; dissection is stressed, which reduces the whole to its parts. During the clinical years, patients are viewed as disease entities rather than people. Throughout training, the student is overwhelmed by the amount of material that must be learned, which heightens the need for specialization. Third, there is an institutionalization effect in the training that takes place in modern hospitals, where students are taught to see patients as hospital cases; the functioning of the institution becomes more important than the individual patient. The result is that a medical school education produces a highly technically trained physician who is able to deal with a diseased kidney or liver, but who may not be able to deal with the person who has these diseased organs (Bloom, Note 5).

There is little likelihood that medical education will produce compassionate doctors if the format of that education remains the same. As one medical student said, for example, about doing an autopsy: "When I see a lung, I concentrate on its structure. I don't picture its being someone who was once living, breathing, and talking" (Fox, Note 6).

Although medical education is beginning to change, with some pioneering patient-centered programs such as the New Pathways program at Harvard Medical School, most medical education on treatment of the dying patient, for whom caring is more important than curing, is still generally inadequate. One important study of medical students' training for dealing with death found that although students begin their schooling with an idealized view of the doctor's role as a compassionate protector of the patient from death, they gradually became more involved with the technical and scientific aspects of medical work and more detached from the patient as a whole human being. By the time the students began to work with patients in the third year, "early experiences with dying patients make clear the necessity of detaching oneself from the emotional trauma of death." To do this, the students tended to define patients as scientific entities, and to deal with the pieces of the organism rather than the whole person (Coombs and Powers, Note 7).

The following example demonstrates this view of the patient. "A 64-year-old woman died of gastrointestinal carcinoma. Her dying had been slow and in many ways difficult because of confusional periods, severe bed sores that were difficult to control, and marked nausea. But, through the six weeks that she was a patient on the unit, she was uncomplaining and warm, and several of the nurses involved in her care developed strong positive feelings for her. Immediately after the patient was pronounced dead, the fourth-year medical student who was involved with her care went to the nursing station and asked for an endotracheal tube because he wished to practice endotracheal tube placement. The nurse at the station, who had been on the unit for five years, refused to give him the tube and in the ensuing argument, accused the student of being inhuman, of using the patient as his plaything. The medical student, a sensible and capable young man, retreated, bewildered by the outburst" (Krant and Sheldon, Note 8).

Some physicians, after they graduate and gain more experience, apparently go through two more stages in their approach to dying patients. First, they may begin to question the medical model that glorifies the science of medicine (knowledge of the disease processes) at the expense of the art of medicine (the interpersonal abilities). They may also come to question whether death is the enemy, especially after seeing the extremes to which some physicians may go to keep someone alive. If the physician does not go through this stage, the individual may develop a "God complex" and try to control death by demonstrating clinical mastery over it.

Second, a final stage is reached when physicians realize that to deal with patients' feelings, they must begin to deal with their own personal feelings. However, little evidence exists that physicians are likely to reach this stage. In fact, much of the evidence would lead to the opposite conclusion (Schulz and Aderman, Note 9).

Death education could help medical students reach these last developmental stages. Those physicians who have taken courses in death and dying have been found to have more positive attitudes toward dying patients, and to relate better to them than those who have not taken such a course. While most medical schools include some death education in their curriculum, very few offer a complete course in death education. Although it is encouraging that medical schools are recognizing the need for some death education, the majority of physicians are still not being adequately prepared to deal with death and dying.

COMMUNICATION BETWEEN NURSES AND PHYSICIANS

In the care of seriously or terminally ill patients, the communication between nurses and physicians literally can be a matter of life or death. Research on treatment courses and outcomes of patients in intensive care units indicate that involvement and interaction of critical care personnel can directly influence patient outcomes. Thus, it is crucial to see how such communication may be improved.

Nursing and medical students receive their professional education in separate schools. They may graduate without having had much interaction with each other's professions and each may hold a stereotyped view of the other's role. Perhaps the most important factor in poor physician-nurse relationships is the lack of understanding of the other's problems. This lack of understanding leads to difficulties among physicians, nurses, and other caregivers in working together with terminally ill patients. While a team approach to care is often used, it appears that most of the stress reported by caregivers is related to difficulties with colleagues and within institutional hierarchies.

In exploring six characteristics that influence and delineate team functioning—goals or tasks, role expectations, decision making, communication patterns, leadership, and norms—one study revealed little congruence between the professional norms, goals, and perceptions of physicians, nurses, and social workers.

- Nurses felt that physicians tended to take charge and give orders despite the official emphasis on collegial team relations.
- Social workers insisted on the confidential nature of their records.
- Physicians sought "quick solutions."
- Nurses felt they were willing to do dirty work, whereas social workers offered nothing "tangible" and stirred up feelings.
- Social workers felt nurses sought quick heroic solutions and did not deal with their feelings.
- There is overlapping in nurse–social worker activity.
- Nurses, social workers, and doctors have different social class backgrounds, different educational status, different social distance from clientele, and resulting conflicts in perceptions and relationships (Kahn, Note 10).

Working at group dynamics becomes an important team function when such problems as these exist. It is incorrect to assume that caregivers from different professions can automatically function as a team simply because they have the apparent mutual goal of caring for the dying patient. A health care team needs training to function as a team, but this is consistently overlooked. It has been remarked that although a football team will spend 40 hours a week practicing for a 2-hour game, the health care team seldom spends 2 hours per year practicing, when their ability to function as a team counts 40 hours per week.

Part of a health care team's training as a team involves practice in communication. Team communication problem areas identified by hospice caregivers included: developing trust within an interdisciplinary team, communicating information, power struggles, handling conflict, "incest" on the health care team, and ensuring longevity beyond the life of the original team. Lack of mutual respect among team members may make the patient a victim in a battle for professional turf.

Professional status differences and respect across professions can influence communication. One study on interpersonal distance among hospital staff on four units showed that physicians interacted with physicians, nurses interacted with nurses, and there was limited interaction between physicians and nurses. One influencing variable here could be the personal characteristics of the participants in the interaction. One study, for example, showed that where nurses have high self-esteem, they are more likely to work well in collaboration with physicians.

True collaboration involves an appreciation of each individual's skills and the continual openness of each individual to role renegotiation and redefinition, compromises, and trade-offs. Collaborative care of the terminally ill brings the collaborators closer to each other professionaly: nurses may become more competent in titrating pain medication, while physicians may become more skilled at listening to patients discuss their concerns. This role diffusion also extends to the diffusion of leadership in health care teams. In true teamwork, no one person has the final single answer; everyone can contribute partial solutions, which taken together form a holistic pattern.

There are several ways to facilitate and enhance communication between nurses and physicians, even before the collaborative-care stage. Professional health care education could include courses and socialization processes that encourage collaborative approaches to planning, implementing, and evaluating patient care. If nursing and medical students were to participate together in professional core courses, they might develop an appreciation of each other's perspectives, values, and goals. Ideally this would continue as they assumed responsibility for patient care. A related curriculum approach might involve student fieldwork with the other profession. One medical and nursing school, for instance, developed an innovative nursing rotation for first-year medical students, to familiarize the students with nurses' roles. Team development is an ongoing process and hard work. The health care professions need to create caring work environments different from the patriarchal, superior-subordinate team orientation that often exists. One approach to this change might be to incorporate alternative principles of power, such as power sharing, humanistic thinking, and decision making by consensus, into the current working relationships.

Power sharing encompasses patients also: their rights to autonomy, to informed consent, to helpful medical treatment and to truth-telling. A shift from the traditional dominant model of power grabbing to power sharing is dramatic, but it is consistent with the egalitarian concept of health care teams.

Another concept vital to the functioning of health care teams is that of mutual aid. Members of a team form a community of caring among themselves as well as with patients, and only when a team provides support and nurturing to its members can it provide adequate help to patients. This need for mutual aid becomes evident when a patient cared for by the team dies. Both family and staff may feel guilt as well as grief that the death occurred. The health care team needs to meet in an ongoing group to discuss the grief and other reactions caused by a patient's death. Regular meetings at which staff are encouraged to talk about the problems that arise and their own feelings will often help provide this support.

To communicate caring, caregivers must acknowledge their own humanity. Caregivers may deny their own human aspects because they feel that in failing to cure a dying patient, they have failed not only that patient but also themselves and their colleagues. Or perhaps the caregiver's fears of death are so frightening that he or she cannot share these feelings. The creation of a caring work environment may give the caregiver permission to feel, and therefore to grieve the loss of a patient. Then the caregiver may, in turn, be more comfortable helping other clients. With the support of colleagues, emotional vulnerability need not be feared but can be used as a vehicle for the caregivers' growth as well as for the growth of the patients.

REFERENCE NOTES

1. MacInnis, K. Making goodbyes. *American Journal of Nursing*, 1992, *92* (3), 120.
2. Weisman, A. Care and comfort for the dying. In S. Troup and W. Green (eds.), *The patient, death and the family*. New York: Scribner's, 1974.
3. Noyes, R., & Clancy, J. The dying role: Its relevance to improved patient care. *Psychiatry*, 1977, *46*, 41–47.
4. Moller, D.W. *On death without dignity, the human impact of technical dying*. Amityville, N.Y.: Baywood Publishing, 1990, p. 35.
5. Bloom, S. Some implications of studies in the professionalization of the physician. In E.G. Jaco (ed.), *Patients, physicians and illness*. New York: Free Press, 1958.
6. Fox, R. as cited in Moler, D.W., op. cit., p.27.
7. Coombs, R., & Powers, P. Socialization for death: The physician's role. In L. Lo-Flano (ed.), *Toward a sociology of death and dying*. Beverly Hills, CA: Sage Publications, 1975, p. 22.
8. Krant, M., & Sheldon, A. The dying patient: Medicine's responsibility. *Journal of Thanatology*, 1971, *1*, 1–21. Quote from pp. 17–18.
9. Schulz, R., & Aderman, D. How the medical staff copes with dying patients: A critical review. In R. Kalish (ed.), *The dying and bereaved*. Amityville, N.Y.: Baywood Publishing, 1980.
10. Kahn, A. Institutional constraints in inter-professional practice. In H. Rehr (ed.), *Medicine and social work*. New York: Prodist, 1974, pp. 14–25.

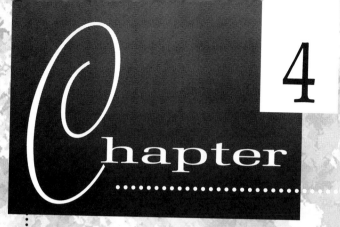

Chapter 4

Hospitals and Dying Patients

Most Americans will die in some type of health care institution. The absence of multigenerational and extended family units, coupled with high-technology medicine and a belief in controlling mortality, have contributed to this institutionalization of dying in the United States.

The immediate priority when dying patients enter institutions is the care they want and need. Many factors influence the provision of that care, including the health care providers, patients, and families and the effects of cultural beliefs, organizational structure, and institutional values on caregiving. It is recognized that hospitals, nursing homes, and hospices all provide significant caregiving for dying patients. However, since acute-care hospitals are the initial institutional experience for most patients, this discussion centers on the hospital.

A HISTORY OF HOSPITAL CARE

The earliest hospitals existed as the healing temples of ancient Egypt, and as the public hospitals of Buddhist India and the Muslim East. The modern hospital of the Western world has evolved from European medieval institutions that had the same name but a different function. Originally these hospitals did not have patient cure as their primary goal. In fact, they were basically hostels for travelers. Gradually these "hospes," or inns, began to provide more permanent lodging for the homeless and the poor within the cities. As many of these indigent people were physically ill, some kind of nursing care, and eventually medical care, was provided. The care was minimal and haphazard, and the hospitals were crowded and unsanitary, so admission to these institutions was frequently regarded as a disgrace.

In the eighteenth century, there were still many people who believed that the only possible place for recovery from disease was within the natural environment of social life, the family. In the nineteenth century, Florence Nightingale's recognition of the relationship between filth and hospital death rates, Louis Pasteur's work with bacteria, Joseph Lister's work with antisepsis, and the popularity of "trained nurses" and their use of aseptic techniques were among the factors that helped to make the hospital a safer place.

By 1890 most hospitals had established schools for nurses, recognizing that the prevailing apprenticeship system of nursing education, in which student nurses cared for patients in exchange for clinical experience, provided an almost cost-free labor force. At that time, medical students did not have access to such clinical experience, but with the growth and development of medicine as a science, medical educators became acutely aware of the need to use the hospital as a laboratory for the study of disease.

During the last few years of the nineteenth century, a new approach to medicine and medical education developed based on careful observation of patients and broader theoretical teaching. To provide clinical experience for medical students and to advance medical and scientific knowledge, it was necessary for hospitals to reorganize their structure to include teaching and research functions. This reorganization, however, did not affect the nursing apprentice system, which was continued. Having a school of nursing remained a popular and inexpensive means of providing patient care. It was not until much later that the nursing profession established its own educational system in academic settings, away from hospitals and the apprentice system. The focus of nursing, however, has continued to be the care of patients.

A turning point in medicine that influenced the goals of the hospital was reached when the basic question asked by the eighteenth-century doctors, "What is the matter with you?" became the question, "Where does it hurt?" (Foucault, Note 1). The latter question focuses on the idea of a cause-and-effect relationship in disease, implying that once these are determined, intervention can proceed. The "cure orientation" of medicine and hospitals was established. Hospitals thus evolved into centers that served communities, for the treatment of both minor and major illnesses. They also became sources of teaching, research, and, for many communities, employment.

What then, are the structures, values, and norms of a health care institution with a cure orientation? The curing goal of hospital care today reflects the American culture's contemporary concepts of illness, that health and physical well-being are worthwhile and possible goals. Illness is regarded as a mishap, something that can be overcome, and health care professionals are expected to help people get well when illness occurs. Americans believe that there must be a way to solve each problem; there is a certainty that an answer can be found to conflicting situations. These beliefs are reflected in the consistent emergence of significant technological and scientific knowledge. They have stimulated many people in the United States to concentrate their energies and attention on the healing arts and sciences. Hospitals, as organizations of people in this culture, also reflect these beliefs and values.

Hospitals as Bureaucracies

Many hospitals, because of their increase in size as well as the quantity and quality of services offered, high client turnover, and tendency toward increased specialization, have become formal bureaucracies, organizations that attempt to reach their goals rationally and efficiently. Professional caregivers in a bureaucratic hospital system are involved in two dimensions of authority, the professional and the bureaucratic. Both are important to the hospital's functioning, but they may also lead to conflicts for the caregivers.

Professional authority lies within the individual, who has the freedom and responsibility to make assessments and decisions about patient care based on professional skill and knowledge. A bureaucracy, however, emphasizes adherence to procedures, tasks, and rules, and the means—meetings, paperwork, and other bureaucratic trappings—can often become the end. Caregivers working within such structures may encounter conflicts between what they professionally assess is necessary for the quality of their patients' care and what hospital policy dictates. A physician may want to keep a terminally ill patient in the hospital for treatment longer than rules and payment policies permit. A nurse allowing a dying woman's young children on the unit to visit may be violating a hospital rule against visitors under the age of 12. The conflict and frustration in such situations are real; the solutions not quickly found.

If the goal of the hospital bureaucracy is to cure people, then what happens to those patients who cannot be cured? It has been pointed out that "the dying patient represents a series of human events where the needs of the patient cease to be translatable into routines and rituals. It is in this fundamental sense that the dying patient threatens the hospital and its personnel. The routine orders, the predictable activities, when applied to the dying patient, cease to be meaningful, cease to be effective, and above all, cease to be satisfying either to the people doing them or to the patients who receive them" (Mauksch, Note 2).

Professional caregivers and hospital administrators can work together to establish a structure that will support both organizational and professional goals and provide the important flexibility needed for dying patients to receive individualized care. The multiple lines of authority within the hospital, traditionally maintained by the bureaucratic power hierarchy, might be melded with the concept of power sharing, which involves joint responsibility for decision making and for acting on those decisions in a lateral network rather than in a hierarchical one.

Care versus Cure

Death and dying confront hospital staffs with uncomfortable ambiguities. There frequently are no definitive answers to offer dying patients about the time and manner of death, what it will be like, and why this is happening to this particular person. Caregivers, who are used to providing answers, may find this vagueness difficult, and they may also feel that they have failed somehow by not doing enough for the patient.

Patients may feel angry because their expectations for help and care are not being met. At a time when they are reaching out for acknowledgment of their uncertainty and fear, patients are often confronted with tests they may not understand and an army of caregivers, none of whom they see more than once or twice.

Much of the care that dying patients require falls into categories of comfort work—alleviating the aches, pains, nausea, and other physical discomforts often associated with terminal illness—and sentimental work—recognizing the patient as a sentient human being (Strauss et al., Note 3). This type of caring work is not valued as highly as medical-technological work. In the achievement-oriented culture of the United States, not much prestige is associated with the task of caring for patients per se. Caring is perhaps also undervalued because it is viewed as "women's work." People entering nursing, predominantly a women's profession with care as its foundation, often are asked, "Why are you doing that? A smart person like you should be a doctor!"

The question reflects the values and status of care versus cure. In one study of hospital care, for instance, it was found that the orientation of medical treatment was overwhelmingly toward the cure end of the care-cure continuum, despite the fact that the majority of patients in the study had conditions labeled by their physicians as terminal and had been designated to receive no cardiopulmonary resuscitation (CPR). It has been noted that while dying patients in the modern hospital are in an environment ideally suited for the pursuit of knowledge and cure, hospital technology and its values run counter to the holistic concept of the person. Personal and humane care can be given in such hospitals, but those who give such care must often struggle with a technical, depersonalized work structure.

The differences in value emphasis between care work and cure work are not only those of ethics, technology, and orientation to work; there are also differences in the financial reimbursement to the institution for patient services. The practice of predetermined reimbursement for health care based on established diagnostic categories (diagnosis-related groups, DRGs) has fostered profit-oriented corporate hospital care that emphasizes efficiency of operation and a patient-as-product orientation to services. Obviously, there are no DRGs for comfort and sentimental work. Indeed, such work may not be seen as professional work at all but as the obligation of the family. Financial rewards for the institution and organizational rewards for staff come from effectiveness and efficiency in the technological work directed toward cure. With this emphasis, the human experience of dying becomes less important than the technological order in which it occurs. While care and cure in hospitals need not be mutually exclusive, so long as cure work gets higher priority, higher status, and greater rewards it will remain the primary emphasis for the staff and the organization. As a result, dying patients and their family on the one hand, and the staff on the other, may have different perspectives in regard to treatment goals and trajectories.

ROLE EXPECTATIONS

For each position (patient, nurse, doctor, aide, social worker) in a social organization (such as a hospital), there are expectations for the person in that position and how that person is supposed to behave. These expectations include the rights, privileges, obligations, and duties that go with the position. This combination of expectations for a position constitutes the role that that person is expected to play in the organization. Examples of role expectations in a hospital setting include patients follow doctors' orders; nurses administer medications; aides make beds; social workers talk to families and assist in after-care planning. Conflicts may arise when individuals' ideas about fulfilling their roles do not coincide with expectations: patients may disagree with doctors' orders; nurses may ask patients to administer their own medications. Such conflicts can lead to the further clarification, understanding, and development of roles, or they can result in an impasse among participants, with a possible detriment to patient care.

Society has created a special role for sick people. Role expectations for those who are ill include the right to be dependent, to accept help from strangers, and to expect to be helped. People who are ill in a hospital are expected to conform to the rules and regulations of its bureaucratic structure. In one study of a large medical center's functioning, it was found that "between admission to and discharge from the hospital, the patients were subject to the orders of the staff. They were separated from their families. Their street clothes were shed. They were assigned to beds, given numbers, and dressed in bedroom apparel. They had to permit strangers access to the most intimate parts of their bodies. Their diet was controlled, as were the hours of their days and nights, the people they saw, and the times they saw them. They were bathed, fed, and questioned; they were ordered or forbidden to do specified things. As long as they were in the hospital they were not considered self-sufficient adults" (Duff and Hollingshead, Note 4).

There are also behavioral expectations for the dying patient: that the dying person will continue to wish to live, make use of available supportive measures and persons, decrease dependence on the physician, accept loss of freedom and privileges, cooperate with the rules and routines of caregivers, and maintain independent functioning to the limit of his or her abilities. Expected rights of dying patients include their right to be cared for in an appropriate setting by personnel who regard their needs as having a high priority.

The Patient's Role

Once people enter the hospital as patients, they lose their normal social roles and must learn to interact in a totally new and alien environment. Patients need to learn what questions to ask of whom; to do this, they must understand the division of labor in the hospital and the staff status hierarchy. (Questions about prognosis will most likely be answered by doctors; nurses will respond to questions about hospital policy and rules; nurses' aides will give the most realistic information about the ward routine and how things really get done.) Patients will also need to learn the jargon of the hospital before they can understand what is expected of them in this new role. For example, if a patient is simply told that she or he may have pain medication "prn," the patient may have no idea that this means pain medication is available as needed.

Patients from countries other than the United States may well have their own cultural role behaviors associated with illness and may have no idea what their role expectations are in this country. If they do not learn and follow their role expectations, caregivers who expect these patients to conform to established sick or dying role behaviors may consider them to be complainers, to be noncompliant, or to be attention-seekers. Patients for whom English is a second language may be at particular risk for misunderstanding established treatment protocols and for being misunderstood by caregivers. However, as one patient explained to a nurse, "Just because I'm from a foreign country and have an accent, doesn't mean that I'm dumb!"

Patients' role expectations may also be related to perceptions of where and how they "fit" into the hospital's priorities. This may influence how their care is given and received. Do caregivers perceive dying patients entering the hospital as being at the top of the totem pole, as important people for whom professional resources should be mobilized to assist them physically and emotionally? Or are such patients at the bottom of the system's patient hierarchy—people who should do as they are told and who will receive services as directed by staff? While hospital staff ideally believe that concern for the Patient (with a capital *P*) as a total person is the mainstay of their practice, in reality the individual patient tends to remain an object or a case. Thus, the patient is not seen as an ill person in a strange environment, frequently in a state of physical and mental powerlessness, struggling to maintain autonomy, identity, and respect; instead the patient's role expectation, from the hospital's perspective, is to be someone to be "managed," as one would manage a thing not a human being.

The following letter written by a patient to hospital staff summarizes the situation quite candidly.

2:00 A.M.

12 December 79

To all who care about patients:

1979, for me, was a year filled with much pain and agony, trauma and shock, sadness and hurt, setbacks, recoveries, happiness, and hope. I've overdone my time here at the hospital. . . . I was admitted with lower body pains and as a result of an overactive spinal tumor and many complications I'm now a paraplegic. I spent a wonderful month of October at home for the first time since November '78 only to have to return to the hospital again. Hopefully I'll be honorably and permanently discharged next week and with some home physical therapy and outpatient chemotherapy, I aim to stay there for a while.

Enough history, though I hope just the right amount to sufficiently prove that I've had ample experience in the role of patient. Speaking medically, I was well taken care of by many competent doctors and outstanding nurses, though many isolated incidents irreparably tarnished the view of doctor as omnipotent and patient (me) as blind obeyer. I started asking many questions, getting unsatisfactory or evasive answers, and then finally learning the truth, which generally was not pleasant. . . .

I still question; I still complain; and I grieve over what I think is one of the WORST problems in this hospital and probably in other large institutions . . . that patients are looked at and treated by many just as Case #16, Disease #12, Temperature 38. Do you know what it feels like to wake up to 12 pairs of eyes (rounds) staring at you in the morning, or one pair shaking you awake at 2:00

A.M. and in both cases, "and how are you today?" In one case, I don't know yet as I was sleeping; in the other, it had taken me an hour to finally fall asleep and what am I supposed to say now?! Ever have a hematoma (black and blue in street language) on your arm, a foot long, and they still insist on taking blood from the same place? Ever been emotionally upset, drained about surgery, and then going through ups and downs of rescheduling and canceling? not to mention the anxiety of the families too? It's all happened, that and more, again and again, to me!! There's a problem here that many forget, that PATIENTS ARE PEOPLE, TOO! . . . like any other people, except we're suffering in some way and that makes us oversensitive and less tolerant. We've no privacy of body or soul; closed curtains don't often stop the uninvited from entering. How many patients know that there is a document stating patient rights? How about some compassion; a smile? Just sacrifice some mechanical performance and call me by my name! Show concern for me and not just for my liver!

Staff and patients may also have different perceptions of the purposes of the hospital that can lead to different expectations about their roles and hospital functions. In one study of physician-client relationships in a medical center, the researcher found that medical students, interns, and residents felt that their primary purpose for being in the center was for education, while patients, on the other hand, felt that since it was a medical center, its obvious purpose was to provide for their care and treatment. Such different perceptions may result, for example, in patients expecting one physician to care for them throughout their hospital stay, while in reality several physicians, in order to acquire learning, may be involved in their care.

In the hospital, once a person is defined as dying, a frame of interpretation is placed around him or her. Staff expectations are not for a cure. Dying patients may be assigned a private room at the end of the corridor, away from other patients and the nurses' station. This is supposedly for the patient's peace, quiet, and privacy, but a closer analysis could indicate the staff's unwillingness to be in contact with that patient. The loneliness of dying patients is often mentioned and indeed they are lonely, for not only are they going where no one wants to follow but also the people around them prefer to pretend that the journey is not really going to happen.

DISCLOSING INFORMATION TO PATIENTS

The hospital staff working with dying patients must often function within a network of ambiguous definitions of what might, should, and must be done. For example, caregivers must consider such questions as to what extent the patient and his or her family should be informed about the illness and to what extent a disease should be treated. Patients also deal with questions and conflict: Is the physician telling me all I need to know, or should I ask about my illness? If I ask, will I be realistically answered? If I get an answer, should I tell my family? Will the physician tell my family?

Family members may ask the physician not to disclose information to the dying patient for fear of emotional upset. When this is the case, however, pretenses about the chances for recovery are not so easy to maintain as the illness advances in severity. Patients often begin to question the more frequent, longer visits of family members and their increased kindness and solicitude, and patients may ask further questions about their illness that evoke even greater pretense on the part of family and staff. Eventually these patients may tire of trying to get answers, and then live out the rest of their lives without discussing their impending death with any other person. The result of such situations is isolation for all the people involved, and the most isolated person is the patient.

The Awareness Context

Whether patients have been told about their dying, and who knows what about the matter, has a definite effect on interactions between staff and patients in hospitals. It is useful to discuss this issue in terms of the *awareness context*, which refers to those involved in the dying patient's situation, who know varying amounts of information about the probability of death for the dying patient (Glaser, Note 5). Four typical awareness contexts have been identified.

Closed awareness: Patients in this context do not know they are going to die, even though everyone else does. Staff uses a fictitious approach with patients, leading them to believe that their illnesses are not fatal and that things will turn out "all right."

Suspected awareness: The patient suspects what others know and tries to confirm or negate that suspicion. Patients in this awareness context seem always to be on the offensive, in that they are always trying to get realistic information from a defensive staff. This is a very uncomfortable and unstable state for patients, and vagueness and insecurity persist in all of their interactions with staff.

Mutual pretense: This context exists when all people involved know that the patient is dying, but all in some way tacitly agree to act as if this is not so. Dangerous topics, such as the patient's death, are avoided. Safe topics for discussion may include chatter about events on the ward, sleeping and eating habits, the weather, social and political events. These safe topics signify that life is proceeding as usual.

Open awareness: This context exists when all people involved acknowledge openly that they know that the patient is dying. Differences in staff and patient viewpoints can be freely discussed. Awareness of their impending death gives patients a chance to bring their life to a close with some control. They can plan for their family, finish projects, say farewell to friends. They can play a part in managing their own death. However, caregivers themselves may have difficulty participating in an open awareness context and in caring relationships with the patients.

To understand the difficulty some caregivers may have in providing care rather than cure or in not informing patients that they are dying, it becomes important once again to go back to the cultural expectations—the role expectations—for the helping professions and for hospitals in the United States. Treatment of disease is expected; caregivers are expected "to do" something. Miracles are looked for instead of death. Therefore failure to inform dying patients that they are dying persists for a number of reasons: physicians and nurses claim that not telling protects the patient from depression and anxiety. In addition, there may be genuine uncertainty with regard to both the outcome and the time of death. Then, too, the caregivers' own orientations toward death are important factors in their provision of care. Caregivers are a part of a society that does not readily recognize death, and unless they make a conscious effort to look at their own attitudes toward death and dying, they may be unaware of how these attitudes influence their care of dying patients.

INFLUENCES ON PATIENT CARE

It has been shown that in emergency room situations there is a rather strong relationship between the age, social background, and perceived moral character of patients and the amount of effort that is made to attempt revival when clinical death signs are detected. For example, the older patients are, the more likely it is that tentative death will be accepted without resuscitation. Attempts to resuscitate the very young or perhaps the affluent patient may be more energetic. One study also indicated that at private, wealthier hospitals, the overall attention given to patients "initially dead" was greater than that given to patients arriving at the local county public hospital.

The shift from retrospective to prospective reimbursement in medical and hospital systems has pressured hospitals to become more "prospective" in their interactions with patients concerning reimbursement. Hospital emergency room staff may raise the issue of payment with patients and families concurrent with, or even prior to, the initial treatment. And regardless of diagnosis, hospitals are financially rewarded for saving time and minimizing treatment procedures. Such financial pressures have prompted public concern that patients who cannot pay may not be treated and may instead be "dumped"—transferred to a public hospital—or even discharged without treatment. The 1986 federal Emergency Medical Treatment and Active Labor Act, however, forbids hospitals receiving Medicaid money from turning away women in active labor or any other patient in an unstabilized condition, and the law stresses that transfers cannot be based on economic reasons.

Hospital caregivers also may provide different types of care to dying patients based on their judgment of his or her moral character and on perceptions of the patient's social value. Thus: "The moribund patient who appears to be of low social class, is shabbily dressed, unwashed, or smells of alcohol, seems to be less likely to receive vigorous attempts at resuscitation, as will the patient with perceived social deviancy—the addict, the suicide, and the vagrant. On the other hand, the great and powerful—like Generalissimo Franco—may be denied the possibility of an unharassed death and may receive bizarrely prolonged and desperate resuscitation attempts" (Simpson, Note 6).

The influence of social class and status on patient treatment has particular relevance for patients with AIDS, because of the stigma society has placed on them. Ambulance drivers may even refuse to transport AIDS patients. At some hospitals, when AIDS patients are being seen in the emergency room for a first visit, some staff may recommend that they sign a do not resuscitate (DNR) consent form at that time. This can convey to patients a message of treatment futility. Nurses have advocated that DNR orders be discussed with patients as part of their care plan, but not at the initial treatment evaluation, when little is yet known about patients and their responses to the disease.

Patients' dying trajectories may also influence the care they receive in a hospital. Dying trajectories (as discussed in Chapter 2) are *projected* courses of dying; yet a trajectory will, to a large extent, determine where and how a patient will be treated in a hospital. If a patient is admitted via the emergency room (ER), the dying trajectory will be defined there. Patients who are near death may either be treated in the ER, be sent to surgery, or be admitted to an intensive care unit. If the evaluation is that the person may live, care in these areas is concentrated, quick, and efficient, and staff is geared to providing heroic measures to save lives.

Hospital care for patients with chronic illnesses or those with problems as yet not diagnosed have more uncertain dying trajectories. Although they will be sent to medical units more closely geared to providing longer-term care for the dying than in the emergency and intensive care units, staff may still have difficulty in providing this care.

Terminal care may be seen by some caregivers as monotonous and routine. Staff may feel helpless when there is nothing more they can do in terms of life-saving treatments; they may begin to avoid seeing and being with patients. Physicians may disengage themselves from patients as palliative care becomes essentially a nursing prerogative. Often, as the patient shifts from the sick to dying role, the nurse assumes the dominant complementary role as the initial dominance of the physician diminishes. It appears that while physicians and nurses have overlapping responsibilities, the domain of medicine is therapy and treatment, whereas the domain of nursing is care and support. Often when the treatment emphasis shifts from cure to care, patients are even discharged from the hospital.

ALTERNATIVES TO HOSPITAL CARE

If patients' illnesses become stabilized or dying trajectories are established that indicate longer-term care than an acute care hospital setting can provide, discharge planning is initiated. Ideally this planning involves a collaborative effort between hospital staff, patients, and families. It includes assessment of patient and family needs, strengths, resources, and support systems, and it attempts to match these with available community resources if these are needed. Alternatives to hospital care include hospices, home care, nursing homes, terminal care facilities, and supportive housing.

Many patients want to return home and express a wish to die there. It must then be determined what resources are available to carry out the treatment plan, while leaving as much control as possible in the patient's hands. Family or friends may want to care for patients at home, but this may be difficult for two-career families, single-parent families, and people living alone. Medicare may provide such services as skilled nursing visits, a home health aide, and physical and occupational therapy if needed, but once a patient's needs are no longer assessed as requiring acute care, Medicare coverage may cease. Patients must then pay for home care services on their own or find community resources to assist them.

There also can come a time when home care is no longer feasible, despite the patient's wishes. The patient's nursing needs may intensify, or 24-hour home nursing care may become more expensive than institutional care. One common reason, however, is the exhaustion of the family members who are acting as primary caregivers. Nursing is hard work, and it goes on day and night. Months of lifting, turning, bathing, and providing pain medication several times during the night can take their toll. And the emotional strain of "always being there" can be as energy-depleting to a family caregiver as the intense physical care. At this point a nursing home may have to be considered.

"What kind of person puts her mother in a nursing home?" people ask. "How can the family condemn Grandpa to an institution?" Nursing homes are thought of as terrible places by many Americans, and "placing" a family member in one is frequently accompanied by feelings of guilt and shame. Nursing homes and other custodial services are sometimes perceived of as places for the prolonged dying of individuals who have "low social value." Nevertheless, nursing home care may be appropriate when all options are considered.

While many people enter the extended-care facility of a nursing home and only leave it through death, other patients use its skilled nursing facilities for a short time and then return home. Rapid turnover of patients, unheard of five years ago in nursing homes, is becoming a reality. Nursing homes may also offer respite care for families, giving them a temporary break from taking care of patients at home.

Sometimes families' negative feelings about nursing homes are based on the fear that the patients will not be well cared for, that their needs will not be met. Assuaging that fear is difficult, for family and friends may feel that no institution can replace their own care—nevertheless their other options have run out. "Acceptance of what is," can be a helpful coping mechanism to use in this situation. Meanwhile, what many see as the undesirability of the nursing home alternative may serve as a motivator for caregivers and consumers to participate, through professional, community, and political action, in changing the health care system to include more comprehensive terminal care.

REFERENCE NOTES

1. Foucault, M. *The birth of the clinic*. New York: Pantheon Books, 1973.
2. Mauksch, H. O. The organizational content of dying. In E. Kübler-Ross (ed.), *Death: The final stage of growth*. Englewood Cliffs, N.J.: Prentice Hall, 1975, pp. 9–10.
3. Strauss, A., Fagerhaugh, S., Suczek, B., & Wiener, C. *Social organization of medical work*. Chicago: University of Chicago Press, 1985.
4. Duff, R. S., & Hollingshead, A. B. *Sickness and society*. New York: Harper & Row, 1968, pp. 269.
5. Glaser, B. G., & Strauss A. C. *Awareness of dying*. Chicago: Aldine, 1965.
6. Simpson, M. A. Social and psychological aspects of dying. In H. Wass (ed.), *Dying: Facing the facts*. Washington, D.C.: Hemisphere Publishing, 1979, pp. 111.

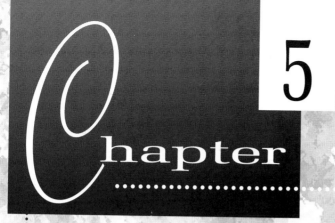

Chapter 5

Hospice Care and Pain Management

In 1974 there was one hospice in the United States; there are now more than 1,700. Hospices have become an accepted part of the health care system in the United States, and they are now professionally accredited, and reimbursable through Medicare.

The hospice is a "concept of care whose goal is to help a person be alive until he or she dies" (Magno, Note 1). The philosophy behind hospice care is to affirm life by providing support and care for the terminally ill so that they may live as comfortably as possible. Hospices promote the notion of a caring community that supports patients and their families so they can prepare emotionally and spiritually for death in a satisfactory manner.

Hospice care tries to keep the patient as free from symptoms as possible, and it also attempts to address the patient's anguish, loneliness, and fears of abandonment in a sensitive, supportive manner. Hospice caregiving teams support the patient's family's needs as well, providing 24-hour accessibility and continuity of service by a multidisciplinary team, which may include a doctor, nurse, social worker, member of the clergy, and a lawyer.

HISTORY OF THE HOSPICE

The hospice concept developed out of the increasing inability of large medical institutions to provide the humanistic and individualized care required by the terminally ill. Today, hospice care echoes the words of the citizens of sixteenth-century England who petitioned King Henry VIII to provide "for the ayde and comforte of the poore, sykke, blynde, aged and impotient persons . . . wherein they may be lodged, cherysshed and re-freshed" (Stoddard, Note 2). Indeed, the concept of hospice care goes back even further, to the beginnings of Christianity, when places called *Hospitia* were run by religious orders to care for the sick, the poor, and the dying. Eventually, with the development of medicine, the *Hospitia* became the basis for the modern hospital: a place for curing instead of caring.

The first modern institution on which today's hospices are based were Our Lady's Hospice, founded in Dublin by the Irish Sisters of Charity in the late 1800s, and St. Joseph's Hospice for the dying poor in England, founded in 1902. When Dr. Cicely Saunders opened St. Christopher's Hospice in London in the 1960s, this became the model for today's hospice care.

A former nurse, Dr. Saunders studied medical social work. While training on a cancer ward, she met David Tasma, a refugee from the Warsaw ghetto. During Tasma's terminal illness, he and Saunders spent hours together envisioning the type of institution that could best serve the needs of the terminally ill. Tasma bequeathed 500 pounds to start such a place.

After David Tasma's death in 1947, Saunders worked at St. Luke's, a home for the dying poor. There she saw pain being controlled through the use of drugs that were not given "as needed" but on a regular basis for the prevention of pain. Saunders returned to medical school, and later, as a physician, she worked at St. Joseph's Hospice, where she studied the effects of drugs on controlling pain in dying patients.

Cicely Saunders and St. Christopher's Hospice

In 1967, Saunders opened St. Christopher's, "a center that would be an ecumenical religious and medical foundation combining the best care for dying patients with opportunities for teaching and research in the fields of medicine, nursing and allied professions" (Hillier, Note 3). The aims of St. Christopher's were and are to understand, properly diagnose, and treat the pain associated with terminal illness and to establish a standard for terminal care. The major focus at St. Christopher's is to assure that each patient is free from pain and the memory of pain.

Dr. Saunders writes about St. Christopher's: The floor plan at St. Christopher's is designed to encourage patient interaction and prevent the isolation that terminally ill patients often experience. The average length of stay is only ten days. This surprisingly low length of stay is primarily due to St. Christopher's extensive home care program. The home care team continues to maintain support in the home as long as it is possible and desired. Frequently, patients enter St. Christopher's for a few days' "rest period" and then return home again (Saunders, Note 4).

Each week an interdisciplinary team of physicians, nurses, psychiatrists, pharmacists, clergy, social workers, and volunteers meet to discuss the patients and to evaluate individual care plans. Care of the patient is centered on the family. Staff often spend as much time with relatives as with patients, and contact is maintained after the death of a patient, to assist relatives in their bereavement. A sense of community is encouraged, and relatives often return to St. Christopher's as volunteers or to attend Sunday chapel services. St. Christopher's also has a playgroup and a school club for the children of the staff and the nearby community. Children play and mingle with patients on a regular basis. This provides a blending of all ages and encourages the concept that death is a normal, natural life event.

The care at St. Christopher's is summed up by the following story that Dr. Saunders tells of a patient: "Mr. P came to us from a teaching hospital with an unsolved problem of pain, unhappy and breathless. He quickly settled to our regime of drugs, and pain was never a problem again. Mr. P used the 10 weeks he was with us to sort out his thoughts on life and faith. . . . He enjoyed meeting students and visitors, and he made good friends in the ward. After Christmas I took him some copies of a photograph I had taken of him at one of our parties. I wanted to give it to him; he wanted to pay for it. We ended by each accepting something from the other. As we were discussing this I held my hand out. At this he held both his, palms upward, next to mine and said, "That's what life is about, four hands held out together" (Saunders, Note 5).

HOSPICE CARE IN THE UNITED STATES

The idea of the hospice was exported from Great Britain to the United States, where the hospice concept was further encouraged by the publishing of *On Death and Dying*, by Elisabeth Kübler-Ross, M.D. Both Cicely Saunders and Elisabeth Kübler-Ross spoke charismatically and tirelessly on the need to treat the dying patient with dignity and respect and on not using the acute care model of care for the terminally ill. The hospice was seen as a constructive alternative for patients for whom continued aggressive therapy did not seem useful.

In 1974, the first American hospice, now called the Connecticut Hospice, began as a demonstration project funded by the National Cancer Institute. The initial program aimed at coordinating home care through a central, autonomous hospice administration; providing skilled symptom control; offering around-the-clock physician-directed and interdisciplinary team service and on-call service as available; providing bereavement follow-up; using volunteers as an integral part of the team; integrating staff support and communication systems; and accepting patients into the program on the basis of health needs, not ability to pay. The National Cancer Institute then proceeded to fund other hospice demonstration projects in Arizona, California, and New Jersey.

Today, there are three basic models of hospice: those affiliated with a hospital; those affiliated with home health agencies, without an inpatient unit; and independent hospices, which may or may not have an inpatient facility. Vincent Mor describes a typical hospice of each type:

A *hospital hospice* has eight dedicated beds in a converted wing of a 500-bed general hospital. The staff consist of an administrator, social worker, minister, nursing director, staff nurses (few aides are used), and a medical director. There

is a limited home-care program consisting of a single coordinator on the staff of the hospital's home-care department. There are few volunteers, and although separate from the hospital's regular volunteer program, they are engaged in similar activities. The hospital's medical staff is divided on the value of hospice care; some are strongly committed to it, while others never refer their patients. Hospital hospice patients have a median survival in the hospice of only 30 days; 25% survive less than 10 days. Most of the short-stay patients spend their entire hospice stay in the inpatient unit. In general, the preference is to admit terminal patients to the hospice ward rather than treat them at home.

A *hospice home health program* is a special unit of an urban/suburban Visiting Nurse Association. It is staffed almost entirely by nurses, with the addition of a single social worker and an administrative coordinator; a part-time medical director is employed under contract. Aides and homemakers, who provide the bulk of care to patients at home, are assigned from the pool employed by the agency. There is a small volunteer program with a volunteer coordinator. Referrals come largely from the agency's existing network of discharge planners placed in area hospitals. Most patients are internally transferred from the regular home health service or are admitted to hospice care at the time of their discharge from a hospital. Almost all have intact homes with family helpers.

Independent hospice programs began as a small group of volunteers, lay and professional, committed to changing the pattern of care for the terminally ill. In time, with the potential for Medicare certification and reimbursement, staffs were hired, and both the number of patients served and the amount of service provided increased. Nurses, social workers, supervisory staff, volunteers, a minister, and a clerical staff now comprise the organization. Plans are under way to build an inpatient unit, but currently inpatient services are provided under arrangement with a local hospital. The volunteer program has over a hundred active volunteers involved in direct patient care and administrative functions under the direction of a full-time volunteer coordinator. Patients are frequently referred by family, friends, or initiate contact on their own. Family support is generally very strong (Mor, Note 6).

Hence, a hospice is not a facility, necessarily, but an organized way of caring for the terminally ill.

Regardless of type, all hospices have some common elements. The unit of care is the patient and the family, with follow-up care offered for the bereaved. There should be home care services in collaboration with inpatient backup facilities. Hospice care should be available 24 hours a day, 7 days a week, provided by a multidisciplinary team with special expertise in symptom control, in which medical, nursing, social work, chaplaincy, and volunteer services are represented. Hospice personnel should also be provided with ongoing emotional support.

Today, the hospice has become an institutionalized part of health care. Its national professional group, the National Hospice Organization, works to promote, direct, standardize, and monitor hospice activities. Hospices are accredited by the Joint Commission on Accreditation of Health Organizations, which provides education and training for its members and maintains an up-to-date hospice directory.

The most important influence on the regulation of hospices is their Medicare eligibility. For Medicare reimbursement a hospice must meet the Medicare regulations on the type of patient they accept and the kind of care they offer. Many of these constraints are quite controversial: for example, Medicare requires a patient prognosis of 6 months or less; there is a 20% aggregate payment cap on inpatient days. The emphasis on home care may limit the use of Medicare to those dying patients who have a family caregiver in the home. The following case illustrates one specific problem in this area. "Mary S is a very independent 80-year-old widow who has lived alone since the death of her husband 15 years ago. She is suffering from chronic obstructive pulmonary disease, a diagnosis for which it is difficult to predict a downhill course with a prognosis of less than 6 months. Her daughter lives 150 miles away and cares for her own family. Mrs. S does not want anyone living in her apartment with her; neither does she want to move to her daughter's home" (Tehan, Note 7). The hospice in Mrs. S' area will not accept her because she does not have a definitive prognosis of 6 months or less; more important, because she lives alone she may need to be institutionalized and may then go beyond the 20% aggregate payment cap for institutionalization. Medicare reimbursement may be creating haves and have-nots among patients in hospice programs, and as a result some have-nots among terminally ill patients may be denied the opportunity of choosing hospice care.

PAIN MANAGEMENT

One of the major goals of hospice care is to free patients from pain and other symptoms that diminish the quality of their lives. For the dying patient, the greatest fear is of terminal pain that "traps the patient in a situation for which there is no comforting explanation and to which there is no foreseeable end" (Saunders & Baines, Note 8).

What Is Pain?

Pain involves emotions and cognition in addition to the physical response to damaged tissue. A workable definition of pain involves the idea that pain is whatever the person experiencing it says it is, and pain exists when that person says it does. Working with this definition, patients' reports of pain are never doubted.

Pain management for people who are dying is especially important, not only because it offers relief but also because "one cannot adequately help a man to come to accept his impending death if he remains in severe pain, one cannot give spiritual counsel to a woman who is persistently vomiting, or help a wife and children say their goodbyes to a father who is so drugged that he cannot respond" (Baines, Note 9).

Pain from a terminal illness such as cancer or AIDS is chronic pain, as opposed to acute pain, which is of a limited duration. Acute pain is a reaction to a trauma to the body and will abate as the injured area heals. Chronic pain, which does not diminish or abate, can range from a dull aching to agony, and it can become the focal point of the person's life. Furthermore, intensifying chronic pain in cancer, for example, generally indicates that the disease is escalating and that death is 6 months to a year away.

Not all cancer or AIDS patients experience pain, however, and we do not have a very accurate picture of the incidence of pain in these diseases. Some cancers, such as leukemia, produce little pain while others, such as bone cancer, produce severe pain. As a cancer progresses, pain gets progressively worse. In the intermediate stages of the disease, 40% of patients experience moderate to severe pain, and in the later stages, 60 to 80% of patients experience severe pain.

The major causes of pain in cancer patients are the cancer itself, the therapies used to control the cancer, and other factors unrelated to the cancer. The tumor itself does not cause the pain. Rather, the pain is caused by the tumor's invasion into various areas of the body such as the bones, the spinal cord, and the gastrointestinal tract.

Perceptions of Pain

Pain is not just a physical phenomenon, for it also involves the patient's psychological reaction to it. A patient's pain threshold may vary according to such nonphysical factors as anxiety, fear, depression, and fatigue. Cultural influences and past life experiences may also affect pain thresholds. These nonphysical factors, which are more difficult to determine than physiological elements, must be considered as part of the process of pain assessment and management.

Sociocultural values may influence pain sensation and the behavioral response to it. In a well-known study of the pain responses of Irish, Jewish, Italian, and "Old American" patients, it was found that Jewish and Italian male patients were very emotional in their responses to pain, tending to exaggerate the experience. With the male Jewish patient, the pain reaction appeared to mobilize the family and physician toward a complete cure, while with male Italian patients, the pain reaction appeared to focus on relieving the sensation of pain. Thus, caregivers' assessment of pain should include an evaluation of whether patients are more concerned with immediate, palliative pain relief, with what the pain means to them, or with finding an ultimate cure for the pain.

Age and sex also influence patients' responses to pain. In the United States, women are allowed more freedom for the emotional expression of pain than men, although this changes as men grow older. Children's developmental levels need to be considered in assessing pain. As infants and toddlers cannot communicate verbally, their crying must be interpreted: Is it a cry of pain, or does it have other meanings, such as hunger, wetness, or wanting to be held? Telling a preschool child that a painful treatment "will be all over soon" does not mean anything, since young children do not understand time relationships. To them, a painful procedure just plain hurts, and they don't see the connection between the procedure and getting well. Among school-age children, there is a fear of bodily injury; however, these children can understand that pain can be limited. Explaining potentially painful treatments and procedures, letting the children know what to expect, and allowing them to ask questions and to express their anxieties are helpful for children at this age.

The patient's prior experience with pain will affect his or her perception of pain. A patient who has had pain that was not managed well will suffer more than the patient who has had pain relieved in the past. What pain means to the person is also very important; to some patients pain may be a way of dealing with an unresolved conflict or with feelings of guilt. Pain may also be seen as a threat to patients: Their life-style or their body image might be changed by pain. Pain may be alleviated in many patients if they understand that staff members are trying to determine its cause, that caring people will be available to help them, and that they have a part in planning how to cope with the pain. Pain may also be valued by some who view the experience of pain as signifying life.

Pain Assessment and Control

Patients in pain will often put on a "brave face"; they may not appear outwardly to be in any great distress and may state only that they are having a "little" pain. It is therefore important that caregivers assess patients thoroughly to determine the extent and severity of their pain. Assessment includes taking a careful history and a physical examination. Taking the history means not only listening to the patient's description of pain but also asking the following types of questions:

- When did the pain start?
- What makes it worse?
- What makes it less intense?
- Do any medications help?
- Does it stay in one place or move around?
- Are you in pain all the time, or does it come and go?

It is helpful to have patients describe a normal day's activity and then ask them if pain has interfered in this pattern: has it interrupted sleep, dulled appetite, limited mobiliby? Interviewing a family member or friend about the patient's pain might also help caregivers gain a more accurate picture of what the patient is experiencing.

Neurophysiological processes may underlie the sensation of pain and should be assessed by physical examination. The results of such an examination may reveal a specific pathology that is causing the sensation of pain and may indicate why the pain is localized in a specific part of the body or why it is perceived as pain in another area. Assessment of the pain may even help alleviate some of the pain.

Assessment of pain must be ongoing, since new pains may develop as cancer metastasizes and the management of one pain may lead to the emergence of a different pain. The following example is illuminating: "An 85-year-old man with carcinoma of the prostate and pain in the right femur caused by a metastasis was treated with aspirin and morphine. Casual questioning the next day indicated that although the pain was less severe, he was still in pain. Further questioning revealed that the site of pain was now retrosternal and epigastric; he had no femoral pain at all. The dose of morphine was, therefore, left unaltered, and the prescription of an antacid resulted in complete relief" (Twycross, Note 10).

Relief of pain should have realistic objectives. The ultimate aim is always complete relief from pain, but in some cases graded relief may be more realistic—such as a full pain-free night of sleep, relief at rest in bed or in a chair during the day, freedom from pain on movement. The latter, pain-free movement, may be the most difficult to achieve, but if patients can rest comfortably at night and throughout the day, their improved morale may help them to cope more effectively. Once pain is under control, continued relief for dying patients is based on preventing any more pain, rather than waiting for the pain to recur and then treating it again.

Pain may be controlled in several ways, including interrupting the pain pathways through the use of drugs, and modifying the patient's life-style. Chemotherapy, hormone therapy, and radiation may ease the pain affecting the cancer patient. Pain from bone cancer, for instance, may be alleviated in 90% of patients through the use of radiation. The caregiver must make sure, however, that the effect of the treatment is not worse than the pain being caused by the disease.

Since pain is also a subjective phenomenon, such feelings as worry, anxiety, and depression may intensify it. Allowing the patient to talk about his or her fears may help relieve the pain.

For patients who want to take control of their own situation, biofeedback may be used. Biofeedback involves the use of biophysiological instrumentation to provide patients with information about changes in their bodily functioning of which they are not normally aware. This information may enable patients to voluntarily control some aspect of their physiological response that is causally linked to the pain being experienced. Relaxation therapy, which may be as effective as biofeedback and is a great deal less expensive because it requires no equipment, may also help patients manage their pain. Relaxation therapy involves deep breathing, a conscious effort to relax the muscles, and some visualization of comforting scenes. In addition to biofeedback and relaxation therapy, therapeutic touch, hypnosis, acupuncture, the use of imagery and distraction, behavior therapy, alleviation of anxiety, teaching patients about the nature of pain and its intensity, and reduction of stimulus are all techniques employed in pain management. The establishment of a trusting relationship between a caregiver and a patient may also help ease pain.

In cases of intractable pain, chemical nerve blocks may be used. This involves the injection of an agent that affects the nerves involved in pain transmission but minimally affects sensory and motor nerves. Results from this therapy vary, but certain types of blocks have benefited at least 70% of the patients involved for up to three months.

Pain may also sometimes be eased by immobilizing a bone or another part of the body in pain, or by having the person modify his or her life-style—by using a wheelchair rather than walking, for instance. However, since this may involve a loss of independence, this method of pain control should be used only when it is necessary.

The most common method of interrupting the pain pathways to control pain is through the use of analgesics. Analgesics used to ease pain are basically either narcotic or nonnarcotic. The World Health Organization recommends the use of an "analgesic ladder" beginning with nonnarcotics leading to the use of narcotics. The nonnarcotics include aspirin, acetaminophen, and nonsteroidal anti-inflammatory drugs such as ibuprofen. The weak opioids, such as codeine, will generally work no better than the nonnarcotics. However, in combination with the nonnarcotic analgesics, the weak opioids will provide an enhanced effect.

The Use of Analgesics

For severe pain, the effective narcotic is morphine. Much has been written on the use of heroin and the use of "Brompton's cocktail," a combination of heroin (a narcotic), cocaine (a stimulant), gin, chlorpromazine (thorazine), and sugar, but recent research has shown that morphine alone is just as effective.

The following are guidelines for the use of narcotic analgesics:

1. Start with a specific drug for a specific type of pain.

2. Know the pharmacology of the prescribed drug.

3. The administration of the drug should be adjusted for the individual patient.

4. Use drug combinations which enhance pain relief. Avoid drug combinations which do not.

5. Anticipate and treat the side effects of the analgesia; and anticipate and manage complications.

6. Watch for the development of tolerance.

7. Prevent acute withdrawal.

8. Do not use a placebo to assess the nature of pain (Creagan & Wilkinson, Note 11).

One new and effective method of pain control is Patient-Controlled Analgesia (PCA). With PCA a patient is hooked to an intravenous line attached to a pump and a button. When pain medication is needed, the patient pushes the button and a small dose of pain medication is pumped into the vein, going to work immediately. A computer controls the dosage and the dosing intervals. PCA allows repetitive dosing of pain medication when the patient feels that the pain requires treatment. It does away with the traditional as-needed narcotic dosing. The patient is no longer dependent on the nurse to bring the pain medication. PCA offers some control and dignity to patients at a time when both are badly needed.

Caregivers' Attitudes toward Pain

Although studies have shown that pain can be controlled in close to 100% of patients, lack of education vis-à-vis pain control and the attitudes of health professionals toward pain can lead to inadequate control of pain in patients.

Caregivers and patients often find themselves in disagreement with one another about the use and administration of narcotics. Patients may feel that they are not obtaining adequate pain relief. Nurses may be reluctant to give regular doses of a narcotic around the clock for fear of the accumulation of side effects that could possibly cause death in some patients. Doctors may be concerned about the origin and reality of the patient's pain. Social workers may feel that no one is listening to the patient's reports of pain. Nurses and physicians may fall into believing that they are the authorities on patient pain, and when this happens, patients may be treated according to the health professional's perception of pain when, in fact, the only authority on pain should be the patient.

Two major misconceptions held by health care professionals concern patients' tolerance of pain and the fear of addiction. Stoicism and tolerance of pain are generally admired in our society. Going along with this is the caregiver's expectation that all patients will respond equally to the same medications. There is an expectation that a medication will have an instantaneous onset and an extended duration of action. Yet drugs have different periods for onset of relief and reach their peak action at different times. Caregivers should be aware of these onset and duration times and should use this information to help patients plan their activity and rest throughout the day.

Caregivers can also have a fear of narcotic addiction for the patient, although it has been shown that addiction does not occur when narcotics are used to control pain. Indeed, "withholding narcotics to prevent addiction may in reality contribute to addiction. The patient in pain who is denied medication or who does not receive an adequate dose may become overwhelmingly concerned with the drug and crave the next dose. This craving disappears with proper administration, demonstrating that patients would seem to crave the pain relief, not the drugs" (Amenta & Bohnet, Note 12).

THE INSTITUTIONAL SETTING AND PAIN MANAGEMENT

The organization of health care itself plays a very significant part in the management of pain, particularly in institutional settings such as hospitals and clinics. Research has shown that the organizational setting for pain management greatly influences the character of the interactions between patients and staff, which in turn are extremely important in the management of pain. The context of the organization itself—its work structures, its goals, its philosophy—affect pain management. An illustration of this may be seen in a comparison of pain management in hospices and in acute-care centers.

In hospices, the philosophy is to help patients on their journey through life. The hospice is considered to be a place where patients may always come for sustenance. As a result of this philosophy, pain management is collaboratively planned by patients and staff to enhance comfort, alertness, and participation in living. Staff members consistently communicate with one another and with the patient about the effects of pain management—how it is working, what needs to be changed. In contrast, pain management in acute care centers may often focus on immediate relief, with the intention of ultimately curing the cause of pain; there is often the expectation that the pain should diminish after intensive treatment.

Balancing decisions about pain is a vital component in pain management. "The pain tasks of diagnosing, preventing, minimizing, inflicting, relieving, enduring, and expressing are weighed with the consequences for life and death, carrying-on, interaction, ward work, and personal integrity" (Fagerhaugh & Strauss, Note 13). For example, take the case of a terminally ill patient in an acute-care center who has morphine ordered for pain relief every 4 hours p.r.n. (as needed). The patient must decide not only when to ask for the medication and how often, but also how requests for medication (a narcotic) will affect his or her interaction with staff and family, whether or not the medication will affect alertness, and how to deal with personal feelings about continually having to ask for help in pain relief.

Components of the staff's decision in administering the medication may include their feelings about drug addiction, the reality of the patient's pain, their knowledge of drug action, and their previous experience in working with terminally ill patients. Organizational and social contexts that are influential in this decision may include the organization of the unit itself—whether it is primarily set up to care for patients with short-term, acute illnesses or for patients with more chronic, long-term illnesses; how busy the unit is; and the unit's ratio of staff to patients. A balancing of factors such as these contribute to decisions about how, if, and when pain control will be utilized.

The following "Ten Commandments" for health care professionals will ensure that patients' pain is well managed:

1. Thou shalt not assume that the patient's pain is caused by the malignant process.

2. Thou shalt take into consideration the patient's feelings.

3. Thou shalt not use the abbreviation p.r.n. (i.e., pro re nata, meaning as required.) Continuous pain requires regular preventive pain management.

4. Thou shalt not prescribe inadequate amounts of any analgesic.

5. Thou shalt try nonnarcotic analgesics in the first instance.

6. Thou shalt not be afraid of narcotic analgesics.

7. Thou shalt not limit thy approach simply to the use of analgesics.

8. Thou shalt not be afraid to ask a colleague's advice.

9. Thou shalt provide support for the whole family.

10. Thou shalt have an air of quiet confidence and cautious optimism (Twycross, Note 14).

When caregivers follow these commandments, patients with severe, chronic pain can be made relatively free of pain and can be permitted to close their life with dignity and purpose.

REFERENCE NOTES

1. Magno, J. The hospice concept of care: Facing the 1990's. *Death Studies, 14*, p. 111.
2. Stoddard, S. *The hospice movement: A better way of caring for the dying.* New York: Vintage Books, 1978, p. 1.
3. Hillier, E. R. Terminal care in the United Kingdom. In C.A. Corr, D.M. Corr (eds.), *Hospice care.* New York: Springer Publishing, p. 322.
4. Saunders, C. Dying they live: St. Christopher's Hospice. In H. Feifel (ed.), *New meanings of death.* New York: McGraw Hill, 1977.
5. Saunders, C. as quoted in Phipps, W. The origin of hospice, *Death Studies, 12*, p. 67.
6. Mor, V. Participating hospices and the patients they served. In V. More, D. Greer, and R. Kastenbaum (eds.), *The hospice experience.* Baltimore: Johns Hopkins University Press, 1988, p. 17–18.
7. Tehan, C. Has success spoiled hopsice? *Hastings Center Report*, October 15, 1985, p. 12.
8. Saunders, C., & Baines M. *Living with dying, The management of terminal disease.* New York: Oxford University Press, 1983, p. 14.
9. Baines, M. Principles of symptom control. Paper presented at St. Christopher's Bar Mitzvah: London, June 1–10, 1980.
10. Twycross, R. G. Continuing and terminal care—Overview of analgesics (historical and chronological evaluation). In I. Goldberg, A. Kutscher, & S. Malitz (eds.), *Pain, anxiety and grief, pharmaco-therapeutic care of the dying patient and bereaved.* New York: Columbia University Press, 1986, p. 110.
11. Creagan, E. & Wilkinson, J. "Pain relief in terminally ill patients," *American Family Physician.* December, *40*, 133–140.
12. Amenta, M., & Bohnet, N. *Nursing care of the terminally ill.* Boston: Little, Brown, 1986, p. 83.
13. Fagerhaugh, S., & Strauss, A. *Politics of pain management.* Menlo Park, CA: Addison-Wesley, 1977, p. 244.
14. Twycross, R. G. Principles and practice of pain relief in terminal cancer. In C. A. Corr & D. M. Corr (eds.). *Hospice care, principles and practice.* New York: Springer Publishing, 1983.

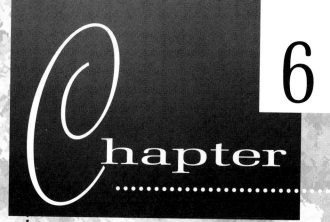

Chapter 6

Children and Death

A child's death evokes inner fears, questions, and anxieties about death, along with the emotional responses of grief, pain, and sadness. Relief is felt for the dead child whose suffering has ended, and relief may also be felt for oneself, that one need no longer invest so much feeling and energy in the dying process. While there is grief that this child will never know the joys and sorrows of a full human life span, there is some solace in the belief that the child did experience the uniqueness of life, if only for a short time.

The loss of a child has many meanings for parents. Perhaps the first and most obvious loss is the loss of the child him or herself, with the concomitant loss of love, enjoyment, and the special relationship the parents had with that particular child. Since a child may be seen as an extension of the parents, as a part of their immortality, this too is lost when the child dies. Parents' hopes and aspirations for the child's future must be relinquished. Another child born into the family never really replaces the child who has died.

Children who are dying also experience loss themselves, and significant changes in their life-style. If they have a terminal illness they may feel tired and sick; as a result of radiation or medication they may experience itching, loss of hair, and weight loss or gain. Family responses to the dying child may change. Parents and relatives may hesitate to set limits with dying children, and siblings they once fiercely fought with may become overly pleasant. These changes add to the dying child's already bewildering questions: "What is wrong with me, and why do I feel so bad?"

CHILDREN'S CONCEPTS OF DEATH

Children's concepts of death develop through a natural maturational sequence and specific life experiences. In one pioneering study, the children involved were asked to express their feelings about death in words and pictures (Nagy, Note 1). It was found that their replies about the meaning of death could be categorized into three developmental stages. Children younger than 5 years old usually do not recognize death as an irreversible state; life and consciousness are attributed to the dead. Death may be seen as a departure, sleep, or as something gradual or temporary. In the second stage, at ages 5 to 9, children personify death, as is seen in this description by a 9-year-old: "Death is a skeleton. It is so strong it can overturn a ship. Death can't be seen. Death is in a hidden place. It hides in an island." In the final stage, reached around age 9 or 10, children recognize that death is universal and that it signifies the end of bodily life.

Robert Kastenbaum, in a 1986 published review of research on children's concepts of death, noted that the tendency to personify death has not appeared in most follow-up studies of Nagy's work. He suggests that "perhaps the world of childhood has changed enough from the time of Nagy's research to replace personification with more objective and scientific-sounding responses" (Kastenbaum, Note 2).

Experiences with death for children currently growing up in the United States can include deaths involving the immediate family and beyond. Children may witness different types of violence, including spousal abuse, homicide, rape, and suicidal behavior, as well as be victimized themselves by juvenile gang violence and violence in the community (Pynoos and Nader, Note 3). The media, primarily television, bring pictures and sounds of violence and death into most households.

Current studies indicate that both maturation and specific life experiences contribute to children's understanding of death. However, much more attention needs to be directed to the unique set of variables, including ethnicity, race, class, and gender, that may be associated with a sample of children at any one point in time and that may contribute to their understanding of death.

Infants

The psychologist Piaget's approach to cognitive-affective development helps us to look at how children, including infants, experience dying and death. The infant's world is centered on the meeting of personal needs: hunger, warmth, and security. After about 6 months, infants become more aware of their mothers as an individual separate from themselves. They are aware of their mother's absence and of when their needs aren't being met, and they may exhibit separation anxiety.

Although infants do not yet recognize death, feelings of loss and separation are part of a developing death awareness. Children who have been separated from their mother exhibit such changes as listlessness, quietness, unresponsiveness to a smile or a coo, and physical changes including weight loss, decrease in activity, and lack of sleep. Therefore, when terminally ill infants are hospitalized, it is important that parents be allowed to stay with them if they wish. (Parents may also need to plan their schedule so they can still spend time with the rest of their family too.)

Toddlers to Age 7

During what Piaget calls the preoperational period of cognitive-affective development (at 18 months of age to 6 or 7 years), children's thoughts are egocentric and magical. Toddlers are very much concerned with themselves and with their ability to do things. They are developing motor ability, self-awareness, and feelings of power in relation to the environment. However, along with these powerful feelings come feelings of fear related to maintaining body integrity and safety. Thus, in caring for toddlers it is important to explain in simple terms any procedure to be performed on them. Also, since separation continues to be a primary concern, parents may be encouraged to stay with their hospitalized children.

Preschool children, developing language skills and a lively and curious interest in the world, are beginning to collect knowledge related to death, and they like talking about heaven, God, and burials. One 4-year-old boy attending his grandmother's funeral asked his father, "Where is grandma?" When told that grandma went to heaven to be with God, the child followed with, "Then who is in that box?"

The child's concept of death may involve magical thinking, the idea that thoughts can cause action. Children may feel that they must have done or thought something "bad" to become ill, or that if a loved one died it was because of some personal thought or wish of the child's. Parents and caregivers must listen for cues from dying children, who may feel guilty about something they did that they believe brought the illness upon them. Dying children need to be reassured that they have not done anything wrong and that they are not alone.

Ages 7 to 12

During the period of concrete operational thought, at 7 to 12 years, children are beginning to realize the finality and inevitability of death. They note that when grandparents or friends die, they do not come back. Children may cope with this anxiety-producing sense of separation and loss by developing rituals to ward off these frightening thoughts, such as always running fast when they have to pass a cemetery.

Children at this age may use intellectual coping, too: trying to find out how things work, or thinking through the cause-and-effect nature of an illness. School-age children who are dying are still developing their intellectual independence and may need time away from parents and hospital staff for this. Maintaining normal daily activities such as school, for even a short period of time, is important to enhance children's self-esteem and to indicate that adults have not given up on them because of their illness.

Adolescents

According to Piaget, the period of formal operations, or logical thinking, begins around 12 or 13 years of age. Adolescents generally have sufficient ego development to understand the meaning and ramifications of death, but the reality of personal death is difficult to accept. Adolescence is a busy time, and death anxiety may be denied or used in new ways to affirm the ideals of life, such as developing altruistic values, humanistic goals, and expanding emotional and intellectual capacities. Denial of mortality may be seen in the adolescent's death-defying infatuation with speeding cars and experimentation with mind-altering drugs. Scoffing at the safe sex practices involved in the prevention of HIV and AIDS and other sexually transmitted diseases may also be a part of this mortality denial.

Adolescents are concerned with their future, with preparing for a career, with becoming somebody. Thus terminally ill adolescents experience great frustration because while they may have decided on their goals in life, they now will not be able to attain them. While adults who are dying have some chance to review what goals they have met, dying adolescents have not had the chance to try out their newly formed values, beliefs, and dreams. The following vignette illustrates that dying adolescents may need encouragement to talk about their anger, sadness, and disappointment. "Glen is a 17-year-old boy with a rapidly progressive neuromuscular disease. Discussions by staff concerning possibilities of tracheostomy, assisted ventilation, and deterioration of his blood gases are continually met with disinterest by him. His parents are concerned by what they interpret as increased anxiety at home. Hospital school teachers and therapists talk about the 'strangeness' of Glen's behavior. An invitation to talk with his primary physician about his depression reveals he is not concerned directly with dying but with his virginity. Sexual fulfillment, previously a future goal, has become an immediate one, 'before I get hooked up on all that machinery' " (Hostler, Note 4).

TALKING WITH CHILDREN ABOUT DEATH AND DYING

American families often incorporate the American culture's denial of death and its inability to integrate death as a natural part of the process of living. Parents may avoid discussing death or showing their feelings about it in front of children. Children can learn to cope with death, but they do have difficulties coping with a family avoidance of death.

In discussing death with children who have suffered a loss, it is helpful to let the children express themselves. Silence about death only indicates that the subject is taboo and does not help children deal with loss. Explanations of death should be kept simple and direct, especially for preschoolers. In discussing death with children, it is helpful to ask the child to repeat and explain what you have just discussed. Young children often have many fantasies and misperceptions about death, and having the child explain what you have said may help clear up some of these distortions.

Children may ask, "Mom, Dad, are you going to die?" and parents often are at a loss for how to respond to this. It is important to find out what the child is actually asking, first of all. Readers may recall here the well-known story about a child asking where she came from, the parent giving an involved biological answer, and the child responding, "That's funny, Shauna says she came from New York!" It is helpful to remember that children are concerned about being cared for and about what will happen if a loss occurs. Parents may want to reassure children of their love for them, and explain what arrangements have been made in case anything does happen. Parents can let children know that they do not expect to die while the children are still young and need their help.

Within a supportive family context, supplying children with explicit information about the terminal illness of a parent will probably enhance their ability to cope with anxiety. If at all possible, children should be allowed to visit the parent during the illness, to enable the child to become gradually aware that the parent is sick and that the illness is serious, and to develop some understanding of death in that context, rather than having the parent simply disappear from his or her life.

Family adaptability and the participation of the children in family rituals associated with death may also affect children's ability to cope with death. Families characterized by open communication and flexible power structures will generally prove more adaptive following the death of a parent than those characterized by more closed communication and rigid power structures.

Children need rituals to help them memorialize loved ones just as adults do, and they can be allowed to participate in those aspects of funeral or memorial services with which they feel comfortable. However, it is important to explain to children what they will see at the funeral home and funeral service before they go there. They need to know about the casket, the flowers, the people visiting. One researcher reported that about 85% of young children who come to a funeral home and see a half-closed casket do not realize or believe that the deceased person's legs are in the closed half of the casket; one small girl thought her grandmother had been cut up because she only saw half of her. Children may not totally understand what is happening at a funeral, but the importance of the ceremony, of saying good-bye and seeing other people who are sad about the death can assist them in integrating their loss.

A Child's Response to Loss

The immediate reactions of children who have lost a loved one will depend on their stage of emotional and cognitive development, but they may include feelings of sadness, anger, and fearfulness. Their behaviors related to these feelings may include appetite and sleep disturbances, withdrawal, concentration difficulties, dependency, regression, restlessness, and learning difficulties. Three questions, whether stated or not, will occur to most children following a loss: whether the child caused the death to occur, whether the child will also die, and who will take care of the child if something happens to the person taking care of him or her now. It is important to listen for these questions and to provide answers.

Children are not as able as adults to seek out reassurance about their grief and to share their grief with others; they need help in doing this from parents, teachers, and others who are close to them. Their lack of sustained periods of sadness may sometimes belie the nature and intensity of their grief; children strongly defend themselves against intolerable feelings that might overwhelm them. School-age children, in particular, monitor their parents' grief or anxiety and are afraid of adding to these reactions.

Children who have lost a parent may have increased physiological and psychological problems if there is also disruption in their routine or changes in their environment. Primarily these children may also fear the loss of their remaining parent. The results of a study of acute parental bereavement in preschoolers indicate that the surviving parents' ability to cope with their own grief and their capacity to provide for the emotional and other needs of their young children were important mediating factors in the children's responses to the loss (Kranzler et al., Note 5).

Talking about Death with Terminally Ill Children

Children who are dying are not any different from well children in their ability and need to discuss death. Children are extremely perceptive and can see through the smoke screen of people not talking about their being sick. Children know from their bodies, if from nothing else, that they are not well: their appetites change, they are tired, and they may not be very interested in anything. Children learn the pecking order and social system of the hospital unit to determine who will respond appropriately to their concerns.

Some children say openly, "I am going to die," while others, less open, talk of "never going back to school, of not being around for someone's birthday, or of burying dolls that they say look the way they used to look" (Bluebond-Langner, Note 6). Although children may not know the name of their disease, they can still learn about it and about its treatment, process, and prognosis. Studies indicate that giving children the opportunity to discuss their fears and prognoses may decrease their feelings of isolation and alienation. The questions and concerns of children threatened with death should be dealt with in such a way that the children are made to feel less alone, different, and alienated from parents and other meaningful adults.

In the late 1960s and the 1970s a more open approach to talking to children about their dying began gaining ground, after it was discovered that terminally ill children are often aware of their prognosis even if they are not told, and that secrecy often sets up a cycle of evasions and deceptions by parents and caregivers that erodes trust in others and provokes fear, withdrawal, anxiety, and frustration (Greenham and Lohmann, Note 7). However, some parents and caregivers still try to shield children from knowledge of their illness in an attempt to protect them as much as possible from the fear of death. While open communication is gaining favor within medical systems, it is not universal yet, and there are still many medical systems that maintain a protective approach. In thinking about what to tell dying children about death, consider telling them only what they want to know, what they are asking about, and tell them in their own terms. It is important to listen very carefully to what children are asking and saying, and to help them articulate their concerns so they can receive help in coping with them.

Talking with children about their dying does not occur in isolation. Again, being aware of the family's culture, religion, and ways of dealing with previous crises is vital. Parents and caregivers need to work together on what is being explained to the child. Parents may need time themselves, to react to their child's diagnosis before they can begin to talk with the child about it. Also, it cannot be assumed that talking with a child about dying is a one-time event. As the illness progresses, new experiences and evidence may alter what parents feel they must tell their child.

CAREGIVERS AND TERMINALLY ILL CHILDREN

Caregivers can offer support to children by attentively listening to what they are trying to express, especially about their fantasies. Children may have many fears based on their perceptions of what they see in hospitals and on what is not explained to them. For example, such statements as "I'm going to give you a shot now" or "I'm going to take some of your blood," without further explanation, can evoke a child's fears of mutilation and death. Depending on children's developmental levels, simple to more complex explanations can be given about the procedures they are going to experience, the medications they will receive, and the proposed treatment plan.

Sharing information with children and involving them in treatment discussions is most important in dispensing with fantasies. With younger children, who often cannot express their own feelings directly, listening to their "play talk" will give caregivers indications of what they really are feeling. A child's comment about a beloved teddy bear hurting, crying, or being scared can tell staff a lot about that child's own feelings. Children's drawings can also offer helpful clues to how they are feeling. One group of children, all hospitalized with leukemia, consistently drew pictures of disasters—fires, accidents, bridges breaking. They were drawing their feelings about their lives ending soon.

The Caregiver's Feelings

Caregivers' awareness of their own feelings and reactions to dying children is a vital part of all their interactions with children. The death of a child in our culture, of which caregivers are a part, is still difficult to accept. In caring for a child with a terminal illness, the staff may feel even more reluctant than when caring for an adult to change from an aggressive treatment program of curing to a palliative one of care and comfort. Anger at not being able to cure the child may be vented by staff members toward one another, resulting in physicians and nurses accusing each other of inadequate communication or of not providing the right care.

Staff members also respond to dying children according to their own developmental level and experience. Young nurses and physicians, for example, may respond with youthful rage, trying to keep death away at all costs and initiating all types of treatment to accomplish this. For nurses who work in emergency rooms or intensive care units, violence and the victims of violence are a part of daily life, and caregivers may become angered by the needless suffering and loss of life that they see. This is particularly true, for example, when a child is a victim of abuse or when drugs have damaged the life of a newborn. When a child dies, professional caregivers and other staff who have had either a long-term relationship with the child and family or a very intense short-term experience may feel the loss.

FAMILIES AND
TERMINALLY ILL CHILDREN

It is often difficult for parents, siblings, relatives, and friends to know how to respond to a dying child, either at home or in the hospital. Children develop their own sense self-confidence and trust from those closest to them; they need large quantities of love and support, and they also need to know the boundaries and limits in which they may live. Children turn to adults for these limits and love, but adults may have difficulty providing the needed qualities.

Some adults may find it too painful to continue to love a dying child. Others, in feeling so much sorrow and pity for the dying child, may release all limits and submit to the child's every demand. In both of these situations children may feel confused, lost, and without hope, for the source of their feelings of safety and comfort has become inconsistent. They do not know what to expect. Thus, it is most helpful if a "business as usual" attitude can be carried on as much as possible with dying children.

Parents

Caregivers must be aware not only of the needs of dying children but also of what their families say and need in this time of crisis. Today's nuclear and single-parent families often do not have the kind of emotional support available in a stable, extended family. Parents therefore may go through the psychic shock and emotional trauma of the death of a child in relative isolation, with little support from relatives or others in the community. They may need some help with the mourning process, in learning how to cope with their own feelings and reactions, both during the illness and after the child dies.

Many parents feel that the most difficult time for them is when they first learn of their child's diagnosis. At that moment they experience symptoms and feelings of physical distress, depression, powerlessness, inability to function, anger, hostility, and guilt. These symptoms may gradually subside, to be followed by a more accepting attitude of the diagnosis and a desire to meet the needs of the ill child.

Some parents at this stage seem to have an insatiable need to know everything about the disease. They seek out extensive information from the hospital staff and compare notes carefully with the parents of other ill children. This seeking out of information may be a coping behavior for the parents, as they try to gain some control in a situation in which they feel so helpless.

In addition to these parental responses, caregivers should also be aware of an apparent lack of affect, or emotion, as a typical reaction in parents. When parents respond in this way to their child's illness, there is a risk of labeling them as cold, noncaring, or too intellectual, when in actuality they are suffering greatly.

When first explaining the child's diagnosis to parents, it is more important to state it simply and directly. More detailed explanations can be discussed later as the parents gradually accept the painful reality. Caregivers can help parents to maintain their control by including them in the care of the child as much as possible and by providing them with all the information necessary to make decisions about various care alternatives.

Parents may often feel guilty about something they think they may have done to inflict this fatal illness on their child. A mother may review her pregnancy and wonder whether she took too many vitamins, for example, or whether she did not take enough; a father may feel he has not been an adequate provider for the child. Particularly affected in this way are the families of children who are dying of a hereditary disease or of AIDS. For families to function in any of these situations, they must move beyond trying to lay blame or guilt, and begin the process of learning to live with the dying child.

Anger is not an uncommon reaction to the impending loss of a loved person. The intense feelings of deprivation surrounding the loss of a significant relationship can be difficult for many parents to express and may surface emotionally as anger, which in turn may also be difficult for parents to express. Parents may turn their anger on each other, or they may become easily irritated with their other children who are not ill. Families may vent their anger on physicians, nurses, and the health care system, complaining about the care their child is receiving. If caregivers can understand that this anger is often part of the grieving process and not take it personally, they may be able to help the family members identify and channel their feelings appropriately, through physical activities, talking with other parents in support groups, or participating in fund-raising activities for medical research.

Fear may be present in the parents' grieving process and may relate not only to what is happening to their child but also to family expenses and income, whether the disease will occur in other children, what other people and relatives will say, and how the family will manage after the child dies. Again, including the parents in planning the treatment of the child can help reduce their fear and anxiety. Caregivers can also help parents begin to cope with the realization that their child is dying by assessing with them the strengths their family has and how they may use and build on these strengths in this crisis.

In most instances, parents facing the death of a child will develop a variety of coping behaviors. These behaviors may vary for parents in a single-parent family; when the mother and father are married versus when they are not married and living together; in a family with young children versus a family with adolescents; in a family experiencing separation or divorce; or in a temporary foster family. In addition, the AIDS epidemic has introduced a new constellation of parents facing the death of a child: aging parents who are facing illness, loneliness, and poverty in their own lives and who are now facing the loss of an adult child. One 80-year-old woman tearfully spoke of her 30-year-old son dying of AIDS 3,000 miles away from her: "I so regret that I'm too old to go and take care of him now. I can't bear that he's so far away with no family."

Parents may develop coping behaviors in response to situational tasks arising as a result of the child's illness. In addition to the need for information already mentioned, they may need to learn to manage their child's illness and death, to assist their child in understanding and coping with the illness and death, to understand the impact of their child's illness and death on all family members, to meet the needs of all family members as well as those of the terminally ill child, and to develop a feeling of control over their own situation (Hymovich, Note 8). Parents may have to work through the conflicting inclinations to fight and run away, to accept and prepare for their child's death while attempting to maintain hope for the child's life, to care for the child while preparing for separation, and to grieve for the child without neglecting the child and other family members.

To accomplish all these tasks, parents will need to trust themselves to develop coping skills and they will also need to trust the availability and capability of caregivers to provide information, guidance, and support throughout the terminal phases of their child's illness. One mother's way of coping with the deteriorating illness of her 11-month-old daughter was to search for information about the disease and, at the same time, to control the timing and amount of information she received about the child's condition. She elected to call the nursing staff herself to inquire about her child's condition when she wanted the information, rather than having the nurses call her on a regular basis. As the child's condition worsened, she gradually began to withdraw and to spend more time with her other child, her home, and her friends. When the baby died, she seemed calm and almost relieved that her daughter's struggle was over (Coddington, Note 9).

Contact with other parents who are experiencing a similar situation with a dying child can be helpful. The primary source of emotional support for many parents during their child's hospitalization may well be other parents going through the same experience. When a child dies, parents can learn that although this is a most painful experience, one does not have to fall apart.

A peer-oriented, self-help approach called reevaluation counseling is one type of parent support group, in which parents alternate between being counselors and clients with each other. Religion and the clergy may also be a source of comfort to parents if they have experienced a meaningful relationship with clergy before illness. Physicians, social workers, house officers, nurses, and morticians or funeral directors may also be sources of support to parents who desire alternatives to traditional psychotherapy.

Hope is an important component of parents' coping throughout their child's terminal illness. At the time of initial diagnosis there is hope that medical technology will find a cure or bring about remission. When that hope is taken away, the hope then focuses on care, moving toward the hope that the child will die without excessive pain to the child or the survivors.

Siblings

The well siblings of terminally ill children live with continual sorrow: the signs of grief, illness, and death are everywhere, whether or not people speak of them. Siblings very quickly pick up on the fact that something is different about a sick child who is dying rather than simply being sick. Children may feel jealousy, anger, and fear toward their dying brother or sister. They see their parents visiting the child at the hospital or allowing special favors and privileges that are not given to other children. Friends and relatives inquire about the ill child and not about the other children. Parents always seem tired and have little time to share with their well children. Family plans must often be rearranged because of the illness. All of these changes may be resented by siblings of terminally children. Siblings may also fear that they have somehow caused the illness and, as a result, feel tremendously guilty. It is normal for children at one time or another to wish their siblings would go away or die; if a sibling does then actually die, frightening fantasies may develop in a child who made such a wish.

Siblings' behavior often reflects these feelings. School grades may drop, and school attendance may be poor. Frequent visits to the school nurse, for example, may indicate a need for adult attention. The inability of many adults to talk directly about death only enhances children's fear and fantasies. When the ill child has died, siblings' grief may be manifested in many ways, including through sleep disorders, acting out, regressing, behaving like the deceased child used to, being unable to separate from parents, loss of appetite or overeating, and depression.

Parents can be encouraged to talk with their children about these responses, and they may also need to discuss sibling reactions with caregivers. Allowing siblings to visit the ill child can sometimes help to clear up fantasies and misunderstandings. Siblings need to have parents or other adult caregivers with whom they feel comfortable and can ask questions, touch, cry, laugh, and act out if necessary. They need to know that they are accepted and loved, and they need to be told the truth about what is happening. They need to be included in the family grieving process both before and after their ill sibling dies. Some families may be able to do this alone; others may need help, perhaps in the form of family conferences with caregivers. Early family-centered intervention improves the health and functioning of all family members when a child is dying.

After the ill child has died, there is often a shift in family dynamics and role relationships. Parents may have lost an idealized son or daughter. Siblings may have lost a big brother, a protector, or a scapegoat. Siblings are also confronted with a new status in the structure of the family. In a two-child family, the remaining child becomes an only child and may not understand the concerted parental attention that now becomes focused on him or her. A middle child may become the oldest child, with new privileges and responsibilities that may be both pleasurable and frightening. Siblings may have to become the caregivers for younger siblings or even the parents. Surviving siblings' interactions with each other can contribute to their own coping abilities as well as those of their parents.

Grandparents

Grandparents are often the forgotten grievers of a dying grandchild. They are grieving not only for their grandchild but also for the loss felt by their own daughter or son and by themselves. They may feel out of control in this situation, wishing that they could offer more help, and experiencing guilt and anger over not being able to prevent this from happening. Frequently, grandparents are separated from their children and grandchildren by long distances, and this, often coupled with their less than optimal physical and emotional health, makes it difficult for them to provide actual physical care or to help with the emotional strain of the child's illness and dying. In families with parents *and* children dying from AIDS, grandparents may even have to assume the role of parents for the remaining children. As with siblings and parents, caregivers can help grandparents to cope by including them, when possible, in family planning sessions regarding care of the ill child and, after the child's death, in bereavement counseling sessions if indicated. Grandparents may want to participate, along with parents, in support groups for bereaved parents such as Compassionate Friends, Candlelighters, and Mothers-In-Crisis.

Caregivers can help sustain families through the child's dying process by acknowledging that dying children have a right to receive adequate pain control, to enjoy unrestricted contact with people of their choosing, to retain as much control and autonomy as possible, and to receive affirmation that their lives have had meaning (Price, Note 10).

HOME CARE FOR DYING CHILDREN

Parents may want to consider home care for their dying child as an alternative to hospitalization, and this may or may not be connected with hospice care. Parents must consider both the advantages and drawbacks of home care in making this choice. The first consideration for home care must center around the resources available to provide the service. One study indicated that problems identified in the use of community agencies for home care included agencies' inexperience with pediatric issues and procedures, inadequate pain management, and reluctance of families to work with unfamiliar staff. Home care services provided by established medical institutions were more likely to provide regularly scheduled home visits by a pediatric oncology nurse, as well as bereavement follow-up.

Pain control can be a major issue for parents in deciding about home care. All the people involved—parents, nurses, and the child—need to understand that pain control is possible and can be effective at home. With the recent development of the computerized, patient-controlled analgesia (PCA) pump, children can administer their own small, preprogrammed doses of analgesic through an intravenous line. This eliminates the need for injection and offers the child a significant degree of control in pain management. This system may not work, however, for parents living in high crime areas where drug abuse is rampant and who are reluctant to have any kind of medication or needles in the home. In addition, it is important to assess what respite services are available for parents who may need to have some "time off" from home care. Hospice programs may offer such respite services, however, as may some community agencies through a visiting nurse service or a municipal social services department.

The advantages of home care include the child's continuing to remain a part of the family—of its events, its joys, its arguments. Familiar surroundings, foods, people, toys, and pets enhance feelings of security for the ill child. Siblings have a chance to participate in the child's care, and some of the mystery of what is happening to their sick brother or sister is removed. The child receives the care, love, and discipline from parents that he or she is used to. This may not be true in hospitals, where parents may feel intimidated. At home, parents and siblings can spend more time with the child, and they avoid some of the problems of transportation, expense, and time involved with commuting from home to the hospital.

There are some possible drawbacks to home care, however. Children may sense that family and friends feel uncomfortable about their dying at home. Some children may feel insecure about being away from hospital-level acute care. The commitment of the family to the child's care can cause some physical and emotional strains. Relatives and friends may not approve of the parents' decision for home care and may make the parents feel guilty for not providing what they consider to be appropriate care for the child.

Perhaps home care can best be offered as an alternative to hospitalization when the following conditions are met:

- Cure-oriented treatment has been discontinued.
- The child and the parents want the child at home.
- The parents recognize their ability to care for their ill child.
- The nurse and the child's physician are willing to be on-call consultants.

Home care for the dying child may involve various methods of implementation. In one common method, the parents are the primary caregivers, with the health care professionals providing support, education, and care suggestions as needed. Nurses may be involved in teaching the family such procedures as administering oxygen, using suction apparatus, and changing dressings, and suggestions as to the comfort of the child, including positioning, hygiene, and nutrition, may be needed and helpful. Parents who assume responsibility for the care of their child may need support in their decision to try home care as opposed to hospital care. They may also need support in maintaining their relationship with their child while experiencing anticipatory grieving. Parents perhaps may need help in understanding that the priorities of children change with a diagnosis of terminal illness. Like a terminally ill adult, a dying child may find the interests and pursuits of other children trivial in comparison with his or her current life experiences; nonetheless, children and parents need to be encouraged to play together and to enjoy each other.

THE DEATH OF AN INFANT

For parents the death of any child is full of grief and is initially incomprehensible, yet the death of an infant seems particularly difficult. The grief of parents after their baby has died is as intense and as prolonged as that experienced at the death of an older child. The pain, the ache, the sorrow felt after the loss of a longed-for baby is so acute that it can hurt as much as any physical pain. One mother described to one of the authors her feelings about the loss of her 3-day-old son this way: "I cannot bear to think that he is gone, that I will never know him as a person, that he will not experience the joys as well as the sorrows of life. I hurt inside—it is like an empty, painful void within me. I long for sleep so I won't feel this loss, and yet it is so difficult to sleep. I wake up and perhaps for a split second life seems possible, but then once more this overwhelming ache, this pain of his death, engulfs me like a wave and I feel like I cannot go on. I will live, but right now that has little meaning for me."

The process of mourning the death of a child is usually facilitated by memories of that child. Families experiencing the death of an infant, particularly a stillborn infant, have few if any memories of their baby, and their grief responses may therefore be inhibited. Caregivers may assist families in developing memories of their baby by providing them with the opportunity to make a decision about whether they would like to see and hold their infant—an opportunity that should be offered as long as possible. The baby's hair, photographs of the baby, a birth certificate or similar items can also help create memories for parents. Caregivers should recognize that parents may need support and help in verbalizing their feelings about the death of their baby. Their grieving can be acknowledged as appropriate and important. Parents need to be aware of the whole range of feelings that can accompany a loss—despair, loneliness, anger, guilt, abandonment—and that these feelings may come and go over a varying amount of time.

Caregivers may have their own difficulties, as well, in coping with the death of an infant. People who select obstetrics as a professional specialty expect to bring life into the world; they may not be prepared to cope with death. Obstetricians may tend to view stillbirth as a serious medical crisis rather than as a situation involving the death of someone's son or daughter. Constant exposure to perinatal deaths produces a tremendous stress on the obstetric staff, and caring for the bereaved parents can be emotionally exhausting. Caregivers themselves may need to learn more about their own responsibility for caring for each other as well as for patients.

Sudden Infant Death Syndrome

A particularly shocking and devastating experience for parents is the death of an infant from sudden infant death syndrome (SIDS), commonly referred to as crib death, which is the leading cause of death in infants between the ages of 1 week and 1 year in the United States. SIDS is the sudden and unexpected death of an apparently healthy infant. The cause of SIDS is unknown, and the death remains unexplained after the performance of a complete postmortem investigation, including an autopsy, an examination of the scene of death, and a review of the child's medical history.

Parents' responses to SIDS are usually very intense. They have had no chance for anticipatory mourning; denial and anger are common. Self blame and feelings of guilt may be overwhelming, and parents may feel they are literally going crazy with grief. Therefore, immediately after the child's death, caregivers need to make sure parents know that their baby died of a definite disease entity (SIDS), which could not be predicted or prevented and for which they are in no way responsible. It often helps to give parents written information about SIDS, and many families may need to be informed about community resources that offer support networks. An organized, comprehensize approach to SIDS bereavement support should include the development of hospital bereavement protocols, educational programs for nurses and physicians, and assistance in the establishment of local support groups in the community.

A child's death affects each of us in a different way; we may feel love, hate, relief, anger, powerlessness, sadness. It may make us look at ourselves, at our own lives, differently. We will not be exactly the same people we were before, as we find that, for better or worse, the child has touched us and we cannot go back. We move on, it is hoped, with more awareness of others and of each person's unique place in life.

REFERENCE NOTES

1. Nagy, M. The child's view of death. In H. Feifel (ed.), *The meaning of death*. New York: McGraw-Hill, 1959. Reprinted, with some editorial changes, with permission from the *Journal of Genetic Psychology*, 1948, pp. 79–98.

2. Kastenbaum, R. *Death, society and human experience* (3rd ed.). Columbus, Ohio: Merrill, 1986.

3. Pynoos, R. S., & Nader, K. Children's exposure to violence and traumatic death. *Psychiatric Analysis*, 1990, *20* (6), 334–344.

4. Hostler, S. L. The development of the child's concept of death. In O. J. Sahler (ed.), *The child and death*. St. Louis: Mosby, 1978, pp. 22–23.

5. Kranzler, E. M., Shaffer, D. Wasserman, G., & Davies, M. Early childhood bereavement. *Journal of the American Academy of Child and Adolescent Psychiatry*, 1990, *29* (4), 513–520.

6. Bluebond-Langner, M. *The private worlds of dying children*. Princeton, N.J.: Princeton University Press, 1978.

7. Greenham, D. E., & Lohmann, R. A. Children facing death: Recurring patterns of adaptation. *Health and Social Work*, 1982, *7* (2), 89–94.

8. Hymovich, D. P. Child and family teachings: Special needs and approaches. *Hospice Journal: Physical, Psychosocial, and Pastoral Care of the Dying*, 1986, *2* (1), 103–120.

9. Coddington, M. A mother struggles to cope with her child's deteriorating illness. *Maternal-Child Nursing Journal*, 1976, *5* (1), 39–44.

10. Price, K. Quality of life for terminally ill children. *Social Work*, 1989, *34* (1), 53–54.

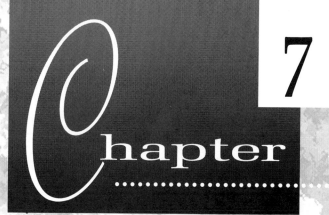

Chapter 7

Living with AIDS

Kathleen M. Nokes

As of December 1991, the Centers for Disease Control (CDC) in Atlanta reported that in the United States 200,000 persons had been diagnosed with AIDS and more than 100,000 of those people had died. Of the remaining persons living with AIDS, some are coping with the terminal phase of the illness while others are actively dying. The largest numbers of persons with AIDS are found in New York, California, and Florida, but absolute numbers do not tell the whole story. When the incidence of AIDS is broken down according to total populations within specific areas, the areas with the greatest number of cases per 100,000 persons are Washington D.C., Puerto Rico, and New York City.

UNDERSTANDING HIV DISEASE

AIDS, acquired immune deficiency syndrome, is the last stage of a long disease process that depletes the ability of the person's immune system to respond to any infection. Human immunodeficiency virus-1 (HIV-1), otherwise referred to as HIV, has been implicated as the organism causing AIDS, but the pathology known as AIDS can only occur when the person's immune system is depressed to a critical level. Then the HIV-infected person no longer responds adequately to infections from organisms that would not cause disease in otherwise healthy persons.

The course of HIV disease is highly variable in each individual. It seems to be influenced by a variety of factors, including the virulence of the infecting strain of HIV, the mental and physical resistance of the person infected, the adequacy of available support systems, and the presence of other infectious diseases, such as hepatitis B and tuberculosis.

The two major routes of HIV transmission are through unsafe sex with an infected man or woman and through sharing drug use equipment (needles) contaminated by infected blood. Between 5 and 15 years can pass between the time that a person becomes infected with HIV and the appearance of symptoms. Approximately 50% of persons report flu-like symptoms in the weeks immediately following infection, but most people do not remember experiencing any specific problems.

The time between HIV infection and the development of antibodies to HIV—referred to as the window period—usually ranges between six weeks and six months. The blood tests for HIV that are widely used, specifically the ELISA and the Western blot tests, only test for antibodies to HIV and

Special thanks to Ray Woolacott for sharing his experiences.

do not test directly for the virus. Therefore a person can be infected with HIV and remain negative on the antibody blood test during the window period.

White blood cells normally provide the first line of defense against any infection. HIV has an affinity for specific types of white blood cells, specifically lymphocytes and monocytes. Both of these white blood cells are characterized by having CD4 receptors on their cell membranes, and HIV gets into these white blood cells by interacting with the CD4 receptor on the cell. HIV is transported within the infected person's bloodstream by activated monocytes, and it lives and replicates within a specific type of lymphocyte, the T4 lymphocyte. When HIV infects a T4 lymphocyte, it becomes part of the genetic structure of that T4 cell. HIV can remain dormant within the infected T4 cell for long periods of time. Through mechanisms that are not entirely clear, HIV gradually depletes the person's supply of T4 lymphocytes.

By examining the T cell levels in the blood, some estimate of the duration of HIV infection can be derived. Persons with HIV become very familiar with their T cell counts, and it is essential that health care providers become knowledgeable about these test results and their interpretation. Two types of T cells are particularly important: T4 and T8 cells. T4 cells are also known as CD4 cells or as T helper cells. T8 cells are also known as CD8 cells or as T suppressor cells. The normal ranges for T4 and T8 cells vary greatly between laboratories and differ between infants and adults, but the normal ratio of T helper to T suppressor cells is 2 to 1. An uninfected person has twice as many T4 as T8 cells, and this ratio of helper to suppressor cells allows the person to resist infection. The ratio of T helper and T suppressor cells in the HIV-infected person reverses and over time there can be many more T suppressor than T helper cells. The health care provider needs to know not only the patient's number of T4 cells but also the ratio of T4 to T8 cells.

Treatment decisions related to management of HIV infection are linked to T cell counts. Clients are started on antiviral drugs to fight HIV, such as zidovudine (AZT), dideoxynosine (DDI), or deoxycytidine (DDC), when T4 cell counts drop below 500. They are placed on medication regimens to prevent *Pneumocystis carinii* pneumonia, such as bactrim or aerosol pentamidine, when T4 cells drop below 200. A health care provider who does not have access to recent blood work can judge the extent of HIV disease by assessing the kind of treatment that a person is receiving.

To illustrate this, we can look at the case of Earvin "Magic" Johnson. The announcement that Magic Johnson was started on AZT shortly after it was learned that he was HIV positive indicates that his T4 cell count was below 500. It is believed that certain opportunistic infections cannot occur unless the T4 cell depression reaches a certain critical level. For example, *Pneumocystis carinii* pneumonia is not perceived as a potential problem until the T4 cell count drops below 200; cytomegalovirus retinitis (CMV retinitis), an eye disorder that can result in blindness, becomes much more of a problem if the client's T4 cells are below 50.

In 1985, the CDC first developed a series of definitions for AIDS; they were revised in 1987 and again in 1993. The 1993 CDC definition of the disease creates a new category of persons with AIDS: those who have a T4 (CD4) cell count below 200. Since many HIV-infected persons have T4 cell counts below 200 but until now have not met the CDC definition of AIDS, the new category is expected to greatly increase the numbers of persons diagnosed with AIDS. While this new category has the benefit of being objective and not based on the skill of a diagnostician, it will confuse the issue of when the HIV-infected person becomes terminally ill. One client with 19 T4 cells told me that he would begin to worry about developing AIDS when his T4 cells dropped to 5—he would wait until then to enter an alcohol detoxification program and would continue his three-year wait for better housing. Another client, recently discharged from prison, had 6 T4 cells and 803 T8 cells, for a ratio of 0.02, and had no AIDS-defining problems according to the 1987 CDC criteria. His major concerns were finding a better place to live and staying drug-free. Neither of these clients perceived themselves as being terminally ill nor did they appear particularly sick.

The CDC's 1987 definition of AIDS was complex but had become familiar to many. There were essentially four categories of AIDS-defining problems: opportunistic infections, such as *Pneumocystis carinii* pneumonia; unusual cancers, such as Kaposi's sarcoma and non-Hodgkin's lymphoma; dementia; and constitutional disease, which consisted of the loss of 10% of the body's weight and persistent diarrhea. Documented evidence of one or more of these problems should signal to the health care provider that the client is entering the terminal phase of HIV disease. Multiple recurrent opportunistic infections, recurrent refractory HIV-related lymphoma, and refractory wasting have been associated with a poor prognosis (von Gunten et al., Note 1). Additional indicators that the person with AIDS is terminally ill may be severe wasting syndrome, progressive decline of the person's mental status, generalized deterioration of all body systems, and unresponsiveness to treatment

THE FACE OF PERSONS WITH AIDS

Although the demographic variables of persons becoming infected with HIV are changing, in the early 1990s the vast majority of persons with AIDS in the United States are men who have had sex with men, and persons of color (CDC, Note 2). While these groups may seem to have little in common with each other, both are stigmatized by the predominant majority, and AIDS is used as an additional reason to discriminate against persons in either of these groups. Violence against gay people and racism increased during the 1980s, as evidenced by the rise in bias-related crimes. Learning that one is suffering from a terminal illness is devastating enough, but this devastation increases drastically when that illness is socially unacceptable and is associated with behaviors that the ill person may have preferred to conceal.

The stereotypical picture of an injecting drug user or gay man is often far from reality, and it can be difficult to tell if a person engages in this life-style. People may not completely report their life experiences. For a variety of reasons, they may neglect to mention their bisexuality or "weekend" drug use or occasional sexual experiences with prostitutes. Particular cultural practices affect whether these behaviors are shared, for example, as when sexual practices expected of men in a certain culture are abhorred in the women of that culture. Religious teachings that specific behaviors are sinful also reinforce secrecy and guilt, and the issues generated by being in a stigmatized group cannot be minimized. In one case, the major concern of an incredibly caring and loving wife of a dying man was that the neighbors in the building in which they lived would somehow find out from the hospice nurses that her husband was dying of AIDS.

Women with AIDS present unique problems. The presence of HIV infection is generally underdiagnosed in women, especially if they do not acknowledge that they have engaged in common risk behaviors such as using drugs or having unprotected sex with an injecting drug user. A woman may not even know that she has placed herself at risk for becoming infected because her sexual partner is not candid about his own drug use or sexual activities with other female and male partners. Women with HIV infection complain of severe and persistent vaginal infections, especially with the *Candida* organism, but this infection is not considered by the CDC to be an indicator disease for AIDS. Women with HIV infection may thus be severely ill yet may not meet the criteria for an AIDS diagnosis. Since entitlements, such as increased Medicaid allotments and nutritional supplements, may be tied to a diagnosis of AIDS, women who are severely ill from HIV disease often do not receive the same benefits as men with AIDS. The new CDC criteria that create an AIDS-diagnosis category for those with fewer than 200 T4 cells attempt to address this issue. The Social Security Administration is responding to this potential change in the criteria by moving away from linking entitlements to an AIDS diagnosis.

Women are also specially affected by AIDS because as mothers they are often the primary caregiver for an adult or child who is dying of AIDS. A not uncommon picture is that of a family in which the man is dying of AIDS and the woman is coping with being HIV infected herself while caring for her husband—and sometimes young children who also have the disease. Grandparents, often grandmothers, also serve as primary care-givers for their dying adult children and grandchildren of varying ages. The financial and emotional strain that this situation imposes on the grandparents cannot be underestimated.

HEALTH CARE CONCERNS OF PERSONS WITH AIDS

The person with AIDS experiences many milestones during the course of the illness, including starting antiviral medications, taking medications to prevent *Pneumocystis carinii* pneumonia, and finally being diagnosed not with HIV infection but with full-blown AIDS. Persons with AIDS experience ambiguous feelings, because there is an uncertainty about death that goes along with an unclear prognosis. Since HIV is a relatively new infectious disease, there is always a hope that the cure will be discovered just in time or that a new drug will become available that will stop the deterioration and prolong life. The uneven course of AIDS, reports of long-term survivors, the lack of standardized medical treatments, and a chaotic health care system all add to the ambiguity. Some clients embrace alternative or complementary therapies such as homeopathy and taking mega-doses of vitamins; their partners may even become concerned that they may be harming themselves by going on a "health binge," especially if the person with AIDS refuses to integrate more standardized interventions. The dying trajectory is different for each person with AIDS, and certain critical junctures within this trajectory are not clearly established.

In a study of the amount of psychosocial support required by patients with AIDS compared with non-AIDS hospice patients of the same average age, it was found that AIDS patients required significantly more psychosocial support than non-AIDS patients. Persons with AIDS have multiple concerns that include locating appropriate health care, dealing with numerous losses, trying to plan for an uncertain future, pain, and physical deterioration.

Technology actually sorely limits access to health care for persons with AIDS. The benefit of such medical technology as parenteral nutrition or hyperalimentation to control the weight loss, for example, is often outweighed by the risks of causing an overwhelming systemic infection from the intravenous equipment. Many of the drugs used to treat the opportunistic infections, such as Foscarnet for CMV retinitis, require extensive hydration, intravenous access, and careful monitoring, all of which are not available to all AIDS patients.

The Financial Issues

Access to appropriate health care is dependent on financial status as well as availability of expert services and technology. Persons with AIDS are often too weak to continue to work and therefore often lose the health insurance that was one of their employment benefits. Medicare benefits for persons with an AIDS-related disability only go into effect two years after the disability is determined—and two years is longer than many persons with AIDS will live.

Medicaid eligibility differs from state to state, and it requires patience and skill to get access to it. The individual's own financial resources will need to be depleted before Medicaid is approved; this process is known as "spending down." The person must first have spent any savings and liquidated any property to meet the rather stringent Medicaid criteria. In some states, a person can collect on a preexisting life insurance policy to delay complete exhaustion of resources. The process of applying for entitlements can be particularly difficult for a person who has always been financially self-sufficient, and the long waiting periods in crowded offices can be especially stressful for a person who feels physically ill and may be experiencing frequent bouts of diarrhea. For the person with AIDS recently discharged from prison, where he or she was receiving health care, the gap in continuity of treatment necessitated by waiting until Medicaid is reactivated is very frustrating.

Getting Expert Treatment

Even when persons with AIDS have sufficient financial resources, they may not have access to expert health care providers. Because the treatment of HIV disease changes almost daily, health care providers must continually update themselves about how to tailor their clients' treatment. Medicaid clients being treated by an HIV-specific interdisciplinary health care team within an inner-city clinic may receive more up-to-date treatment than clients paying out of pocket for private medical care from providers who have few HIV-infected clients in their caseload. The person with AIDS needs reassurance that different plans of care result from advances in understanding about how to treat HIV disease, and not necessarily from confusion.

The prescribed treatment plan for *Pneumocystis carinii* pneumonia is a good illustration of this point. Initially, regular dose bactrim was prescribed, but almost half of those taking it developed a troublesome skin rash. Aerosol pentamidine was then prescribed as the preferred treatment, but it was found that this intervention did not work as well as bactrim, so bactrim again became the preferred treatment, at lower doses. When a health care team treats only one to two AIDS clients a week, it is difficult to stay abreast of the latest shifts in treatment.

Limited resources are also a factor in even determining whether a person is HIV infected. Unless a client is involved in a research study or can pay out of pocket for special blood tests for HIV, only antibody testing for the virus is available. This lack of access to direct viral testing is a particular problem for HIV-positive mothers. Virtually all babies born of HIV-infected mothers will be positive on the HIV antibody test. These positive test results are very difficult to interpret, however, because it is not known whether the antibodies that are causing the baby to be positive on the blood test come from the mother or are being produced by the baby who is actually infected with HIV. Although technology exists to test a person's blood for the virus directly, it is not readily available. A mother with AIDS may die before learning whether her 8-month-old son is HIV positive on the ELISA HIV antibody blood test because he has his mother's antibodies or because he is actually infected with HIV.

Facing Multiple Losses

Persons with AIDS are coping with numerous losses. Friends, other family members including children, and a sexual partner may have already died from AIDS. The person with AIDS is losing dreams of living a long life, seeing children grow up, finishing school, becoming a famous lawyer, staying off drugs (Nokes and Carver, Note 3). The mother with AIDS loses her infant child, and the infected gay man loses the love of his life at a time when his heart is already breaking. The health care provider cannot keep the person with AIDS from learning about the last stages of the illness. Sometimes the client knows more about the prognosis of AIDS than the health care provider, and will react negatively if the provider tries to create an unrealistically optimistic picture.

Persons with AIDS are concerned about planning for an uncertain future. Gay men, because the significant relationships in their life may not be recognized legally, have concerns about how different people will react after their death. Helping persons with AIDS to complete tasks such as making out a will, contacting estranged family, establishing advance directives such as a health care proxy or living will, planning guardianship of minor children, and perhaps prearranging the funeral may help them feel calmer about the future. As one surviving partner of a person who died from AIDS said: "It really must be impressed upon people to make a will. Even when all is 'cut and dried,' the sudden interest from previously disinterested family members was rather upsetting."

Pain and Deterioration

There are many causes of pain from AIDS-related problems, and uncontrolled pain is frightening for anyone. Persons with a history of illegal drug use may have the additional fear they they will not get adequate levels of analgesics because of health care providers' own value judgments about giving narcotic analgesics to chronic drug users. Because of his history of illegal drug use, one client with acute pain was denied any analgesic other than Tylenol (acetaminophen) for a herpes zoster infection that eventually caused blindness. Health care providers familiar with the latest trends in treatment of HIV disease often lack knowledge of basic principles of pain management. These providers may prefer to refer the person with AIDS to a hospice for pain management, but these referrals can be hindered by hospice policies related to financial constraints, do-not-resuscitate orders, and the need for a primary caregiver.

The chronic intractable diarrhea, blindness, and neurological deficits associated with terminal AIDS cause intense body image changes and physical deterioration. Chronic intractable diarrhea in persons with AIDS is often resistant to most standardized treatments and requires unique approaches. Kaposi's sarcoma, which is a form of cancer, can be incredibly disfiguring; persons with Kaposi's sarcoma develop multiple skin lesions that vary according to the person's skin color but are often bluish-brown in appearance. Countless case studies of handsome young men who died shrunken and aged from AIDS fill the literature.

At this final stage of illness, hospice care seems the most appropriate alternative. Those involved in this decision may be ambivalent, however. The client, often exhausted by fighting endless battles against innumerable infections, may still be reluctant to admit defeat. The referring health care providers may be having trouble coping with yet another treatment failure. The hospice personnel may be debating as to whether an HIV-related treatment, such as an antiviral drug, has a curative or palliative intent, and if it should be continued after the client is on the hospice program.

CONCERNS OF FAMILIES AND LOVED ONES

The gay man with AIDS often has both a family of origin with biological roots and a social family of choice, which often consists of other gay men and lesbians. Persons with a history of injecting drug use also have families of origin and those of choice: biological relations and drug-sharing friends. The sexual partners of bisexual men and injecting drug users often identify with more of a nuclear family pattern. The diagnosis of AIDS in a family member produces a crisis in any of these family systems. Preexisting stresses in relationships are often exacerbated as roles change, and the person with AIDS grows increasingly dependent on whomever will provide care.

As functional dependency increases and the person with AIDS becomes weaker, the primary caregiver often takes more control over the situation and may exclude others. In one case, Ray and Jim lived together in a rural setting in Wales for 16 years. Jim's parents lived close by, were disapproving of the gay relationship, and made their feelings very clear at every opportunity. When Jim, who was an airline steward, was confined to bed and suffering from growing blindness and increasing cognitive impairment, Ray provided his care. As Jim's dependency grew, Ray grew clearer in his ability to make decisions for Jim, despite the disruptive influence of Jim's parents. After Jim's death, the strain between Jim's parents and Ray worsened, and the grieving process was delayed for all by their failure to resolve important issues. In a situation like this, involvement in a bereavement group may help to resolve feelings of anger and resentment.

In a study asking people to describe their experiences in losing a lover to AIDS, isolation and disconnectedness, emotional confusion, and acceptance and denial emerged as the three main categories of response (Sowell et al., Note 4). The first category included themes of isolation from their own family, their lover's family, friends, and self. Themes of guilt, loneliness, anger, and ambivalence emerged from the category of emotional confusion. Survivors may have to cope not only with their own HIV illness but also with their ambivalence about surviving and forming new relationships. Social support was a significant factor, as all respondents described feelings of isolation and loneliness following the loss of their lover when they had very limited social support.

When the injecting drug user with AIDS becomes too weak to go outside, it may be a relief for the family members, because they know that their son, daughter, or partner can no longer get access to drugs. The family members no longer have to fear having their property sold for drugs, answering the phone to learn that the person has been arrested again, or being physically abused by the person "crazy on crack." Often cultural and religious beliefs help support the family as they take the person back into their home for the countless—and probably last—time.

The sexual partner of the person with AIDS fears that either he or she will become infected despite the use of safer sex practices. Sexual behaviors change as a result, and both partners may start to distance themselves from the other because of an inability to talk about this fear. Health care providers are often also ambivalent about helping couples to deal with their sexuality, especially when there are no guarantees that safer sex practices, such as consistent condom use, are 100% effective. When one client was reminded to use condoms, he remarked that something "funny" had happened during the last time he and his wife made love—but he didn't think the nurse would find the event so funny. He was right: the nurse did not think it was funny that he had failed to hold the condom in place during withdrawal, which resulted in the semen-filled condom remaining in his uninfected wife's vagina. For some partners, the person's increasing weakness and the subsequent disinterest in sex is a relief.

Despite counseling of family members that HIV is not spread by casual contact, some people persist in isolating laundry or dishes, and in keeping small children away from the person with AIDS. A few days before one client's death, his father wore bright red gloves when helping the man's lover carry him upstairs to bed. Eight months after the man's death, the lover said, "I felt incensed," and he wondered how his lover had felt about it. When family members understand that HIV is spread by blood and sexual contact, when they are instructed to use bleach to kill any HIV that may be in the blood on the person's clothes, when they are provided with equipment such as gloves to use when touching the person's bodily fluids and yet they still persist in isolating the client, a deeper fear than that of contagion may be present. The health care provider then needs to balance the benefits of having a family member provide the client with shelter, food, and medication against the isolation and shame that the client may be experiencing. Options in these situations are very limited, and the health care provider can serve as a role model by touching the client without using barriers when giving a back rub, for example, or by simply shaking hands, reinforcing the precautions that are necessary and not overemphasizing the negative.

Despite the fact that the first case of AIDS was identified back in 1981, the embarrassment of having a family member diagnosed with AIDS persists. People make up stories about why their son or daughter is sick or dying. This inability to share the details about the illness of a significant family member impedes the resolution of grief. In a study of families of AIDS patients and other hospice patients with terminal illness, families of AIDS patients had significantly more stress, more rules prohibiting emotional expression, lower trust levels, and more illness anxiety than the other families (Atkins and Amenta, Note 5). Support groups in neutral settings—often far from the community where the person lives—can be safe havens. There, family members can express their anger, fear, frustration, helplessness, revulsion, rejection, and guilt. Sharing these feelings with group members who have also experienced them facilitates their resolution.

Even after death, the family may face discrimination from a funeral director, who may want to charge more to arrange the funeral of a person who died from AIDS or who may insist on a closed casket. State laws vary about acceptable practices, but health care providers should instruct family members about their rights. Community resources are also very helpful in ensuring that discriminatory practices are not allowed. Sometimes a simple phone call can result in a total change in attitude, and health care providers need to act as advocates for family members who are trying to cope with yet another embarrassing situation.

Because of limited finances, burial arrangements may be problematic. Veterans of the United States military can be buried through the services provided by the government. Medicaid provides a small amount of money for burial. Some AIDS community organizations, recognizing this problem, have asked people to donate extra burial plots for persons who have died of AIDS who were alone or whose families do not have the financial resources to pay for the desired burial.

CONCERNS OF HEALTH CARE PROVIDERS

Perhaps the major barrier to caring for persons with AIDS is fear of being infected with HIV. While the risk of becoming infected through occupational exposure is very slight, less than one-half of 1%, the possibility still generates fear even for those who accept the low risk and choose to work with persons with AIDS. Knowledge about occupational exposure can help to control fear, but it will not erase it. It is helpful for any health care provider who is administering direct care to persons with AIDS to understand that the major risk behavior occurs during contact with the infected client's blood.

Occupational Exposure to HIV

Three factors need to be considered in judging an occupational exposure situation: the route of exposure, the amount of infected body fluids involved, and the extent of HIV within the infected person's blood. Piercing the skin with a needle is more risky than getting blood on an intact skin surface, but both exposures should be taken seriously. Barrier equipment, such as gloves, will not stop needle sticks but will be effective protection against skin contact with infected blood. The amount of infected body fluids a health care worker comes in contact with may be a significant factor in determining both whether the health care provider becomes infected and how quickly the disease will progress. The registered nurse who died of AIDS in 1991 as a result of occupational exposure had accidentally injected herself with 3 to 5 cc of an AIDS patient's blood. She was resting against the client's bed to stabilize her hands while she drew his blood. The bed moved, she felt herself falling, and she inadvertently injected her thigh with the syringe filled with his blood. The registered nurse in Iowa who has HIV infection through an occupational exposure in 1986 used her ungloved fingers to stop the bleeding at an intravenous puncture site.

The amount of HIV within the client's blood is also perceived as a factor in determining whether the health care provider will become infected with HIV. As HIV continues to infect T4 cells, the probability increases that more blood cells will actually contain the virus. Clients with AIDS have large numbers of infected T4 cells, and exposure to their blood may be more risky than exposure to the blood of an HIV-positive person who has relatively large numbers of uninfected T4 cells.

Because of the legal need to determine whether an occupational exposure resulted in HIV infection, health care providers who have been exposed to

HIV will be asked to establish that they are HIV negative at the time of the occupational exposure. In many health care facilities, the policies developed to address occupational exposure to HIV require that the health care provider consent to HIV testing in the 24-hour period after exposure to establish a negative baseline. HIV testing is then repeated 6 weeks, 3 months, 6 months, and sometimes 1 year later. A health care provider who is negative at the baseline test and HIV positive 6 months later is assumed to have become positive through that occupational exposure. Workers' compensation and other disability benefits are then available to that health care provider. The use of the medication AZT after occupational exposure is extremely controversial, but if the health care facility offers AZT to the health care provider who has experienced a significant occupational exposure to HIV, the drug should be started as soon as possible, preferably within the first hour after exposure.

The issue of HIV-infected health care providers caring for uninfected health care consumers remains controversial. During the summer of 1991, the U.S. Senate passed the Helms amendment, which would have required any HIV-infected health care worker to notify any potential client that she or he was infected. Failure to notify the potential client would result in criminal penalties of ten years in jail and a $10,000 fine. This amendment died in the House, but it should not be forgotten, because it illustrates the attitude of a significant number of persons in the United States on the issue of HIV-infected health care providers.

Exposure to Other Diseases

While the risk of becoming infected with HIV through occupational exposure is very low, the risk of contracting other infectious diseases experienced by persons with AIDS should not be minimized. Many persons with AIDS also have hepatitis B, and the risk of infection with hepatitis B after exposure ranges between 6 and 30%. However there is now a vaccine available for hepatitis B. Herpes zoster is believed to result from a reactivation of chicken pox. Health care providers who did not have chicken pox may become infected if they are exposed to a client with herpes zoster.

Pulmonary tuberculosis (TB) is an infectious disease that results from a defect in the cellular immune system. One standard skin test for exposure to TB is the PPD test. When HIV-infected clients lose a significant amount of immune system functioning, perhaps when their T4 cell levels drop below 400, they often cannot have a normal PPD skin response, and their PPD skin test is interpreted as normal or negative because there is no skin reaction. This interpretation is wrong; the absence of the skin reaction is due to the depression of the immune system in the HIV-infected client. Even the chest X ray of the HIV-infected client may not show changes from TB when the tuberculosis is present.

Health care providers are at risk for contracting tuberculosis, especially from undiagnosed patients. TB epidemics in hospitals, hospices, shelters, and prisons have occurred, and hospitals in New York and Miami are coping with outbreaks of drug-resistant tuberculosis among patients with AIDS (Headlines, Note 6). Within the New York State correctional facilities, outbreaks of drug-resistant tuberculosis were reported in 1991.

Adequate ventilation, ultraviolet lights, and environmental modifications are essential to protect the health care providers from TB infection. Health care providers working with immune-depressed HIV-infected clients must assess their PPD status frequently—every 6 months is probably a good idea. Children who are PPD negative in the household of anyone with TB should be temporarily relocated until the patient's TB infection is controlled by medication.

AIDS is perceived by some to be the health care challenge of the late twentieth century. Health care providers who want to make a difference accept the challenge of working with persons with HIV infection. For them, the risks are outweighed by the benefits of believing that their work is truly meaningful. Persons with AIDS are young, often very educated, interesting to speak with, demand equality in decision making, and are very appreciative when someone cares about them. Health care providers are excited by being on the front lines in the fight against an infectious disease that will probably be cured, or at least prevented, at some point in the future. The work is stressful but rewarding.

On the other hand, a survey of hospice staff showed that they felt that working with persons with AIDS was both more time-consuming and more stressful than working with terminally ill patients with other diagnoses. The health care provider may need to deal with the anger, guilt, or shame generated by identifying with the person with AIDS. Health care providers need to come to terms with such existential issues as their own mortality and recognize the limits of their interventions. It helps to focus on the joys of the present moment. Although the cure is on the horizon, it will take many years of sustained work before this epidemic is controlled. Health care providers need to pace themselves for the long run.

ETHICAL ISSUES

The HIV epidemic highlights the conflicts between individualistic and public health ethics. Health care providers are most comfortable with an individualistic approach, which emphasizes the rights of specific persons. The public health ethic forces a broader perspective, since the rights of the individual are weighed against the rights of others. The issue of notifying persons who have had sexual contact with an HIV-infected client is a good illustration of how these two ethical theories can be in conflict. The case of the person dying from AIDS who wants to be discharged to his parent's home but who refuses to tell his parents his diagnosis is another typical example. In this case, the health care providers need to weigh the rights of the client to confidentiality versus the rights of the parents to protect themselves against certain exposure to bloody fluids.

The economic impacts of the AIDS epidemic on health care costs is great, and financial constraints generate issues of distributive justice—who gets treated and for what. As the picture of this epidemic continues to evolve, the economic toll that AIDS is taking on every person in the United States will begin to be recognized.

AIDS and Pregnancy

Perhaps there is no ethical issue that generates more discussion than that of an HIV-infected woman who becomes pregnant. The risk of actually giving birth to an HIV-infected child is between 25 to 30%, which means that between 70 and 75% of the offspring will not be infected with HIV (Pizzo and Butler, Note 7). Pregnancy does not seem to accelerate the infected woman's HIV disease. Giving birth to one HIV-infected child does not seem to be a good predictor of whether the next child will also be HIV infected. Religion, economics, equality, culture, and a wish to have children all have an impact on whether an HIV-positive woman becomes pregnant and if she chooses to continue a pregnancy.

Society, through insurance programs such as Medicaid, pays for the medical care of HIV-infected children, many of whom require extensive and expensive care over long periods of time. Health care providers need to examine how they feel about women with AIDS who choose to continue pregnancies, because those feelings will affect the formation of a trusting client-provider relationship. The issue of women with AIDS who choose to continue pregnancies needs to be examined in the context of how women with other life-threatening problems that affect their offspring are regarded by society. The contributions of the male partner to the pregnancy cannot be ignored, and the ethics of this situation needs to be examined through the perspective of the relationship of the mother and father.

There seem to be two groups of children with AIDS, those who die within the first three years of life and those who live an average of seven years. The first group is characterized by repeated infections, failure to thrive, regression of developmental milestones, and often mental retardation. The second group experiences more frequent bacterial infections but seems essentially well. Medical treatment for the HIV-infected child continues to develop, and many of the drugs that are used to treat adults are now being used successfully with children. In addition, intravenous immunoglobulin seems to control many of the bacterial infections that affect children.

Although the research is scanty, there does seem to be a tendency for HIV-infected mothers who have surviving children to live longer than mothers whose children have died. The needs of orphans who are left behind when family members have died of AIDS can be overwhelming, and services for these otherwise physically healthy children are not covered by most forms of health insurance. Special programs are now being developed to address these needs, but much more attention must be paid to these children who have experienced tremendous loss and grief at a young age.

Although community resources to assist persons with AIDS now exist in most areas throughout the United States, they are most extensive in the areas hardest hit by the epidemic. The list of community resources for persons with HIV infection in the New York City area, for example, fills many pages, although budget cuts and uncertain funding have forced some of these agencies to close or decrease services. The large community agencies, such as the Gay Men's Health Crisis in New York, have "hot line" phone numbers listed in the telephone directory, and volunteers answering these phones can give callers information about resources available in different communities. It is best to be as clear as possible about the services needed, and expect to make a number of phone calls before an available provider is identified. If a health care provider or friend is making calls for a person with AIDS, it is essential to first clarify with that person the information that will have to be shared with the community resources. Getting written permission to release confidential information about HIV may be required by state law.

The issues generated by the AIDS epidemic are taxing our society. Young people are dying while leaders in government and the health care industry debate philosophical dilemmas. Most persons with AIDS feel tremendous urgency, since their time is limited; others would still like to ignore the problem. On one level there is turmoil, agitation, chaos, while on a different level there is an attempt to act as if nothing is happening. According to the federal government, at the end of 1992 over 200,000 persons within the United States were diagnosed with AIDS. Countless persons throughout the world will have died from AIDS. This epidemic will continue to challenge everyone into the twenty-first century.

REFERENCE NOTES

1. von Gunten, C., Martinez, J., Weitzman, S., & Von Roenn, J. AIDS and hospice. *The American Journal of Hospice and Palliative Care*, 1991, *8*, 17–19.
2. Centers for Disease Control (CDC). *HIV/AIDS Surveillance*. December 1991.
3. Nokes, K., & Carver, K. What is the meaning of living with AIDS: An examination through man-living-health theory. *Nursing Science Quarterly*, 1991, *4*, 175–179.
4. Sowell, R., Bramlett, M., Gueldner, S., Gritzmacker, D., & Martin G. The lived experience of survival and bereavement following the death of a lover from AIDS. *Image: Journal of Nursing Scholarship*, 1991, *23*, 89–94.
5. Atkins, R., & Amenta, M. Family adaptation to AIDS: A comparative study. *The Hospice Journal*, 1991, *7*, 71–83.
6. Headlines: Devastating TB epidemics. *American Journal of Nursing*, 1992, *92*, 9.
7. Pizzo, P., & Butler, K. In the vertical transmission of HIV, timing may be everything. *The New England Journal of Medicine*, 1991, *325*, 652–653.

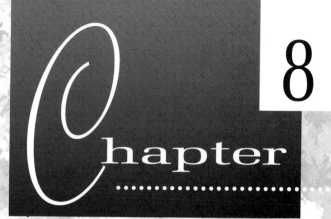

Chapter 8

Ethical and Legal Issues

Ethical issues surrounding death have been discussed throughout history, but because of our advanced medical technology, ethical issues today have become more complex. The new heart-lung machine has led us to question the criteria determining death; there are new treatments that prolong life but have painful side effects; and improved forms of treatment maintain the lives of many who would have died in the past, without necessarily returning them to a full life.

THE DEFINITION OF DEATH

Within the past 20 years, the controversy surrounding the definition of death has changed. In the 1970s, the concern involved changing the definition of death from the irreversible cessation of the heart and respiration to the death of the brain. Today, with brain death widely accepted as the legal definition of death, the concern is whether death should be defined in terms of the whole brain or the higher brain.

Defining death was not simple in the past. Putrefaction was considered the only sure sign of death, but even this was attacked because putrefaction is found in cases of gangrene. The fear of premature cessation of medical care and premature burial motivated the development of safeguards, in the form of mortuaries and legislation delaying burial for at least one day.

As the medical profession developed greater scientific standards, a consensus developed that medical knowledge could lead to the best protection against premature burial. By the late nineteenth century there began to be agreement among physicians that the major signs of death were the irrevocable cessation of the heartbeat, respiration, and consciousness.

In the late 1950s and early 1960s, with the development of organ transplants, there was a push to redefine death in terms of the brain rather than the heart and lungs. It became imperative to define death in a way that would protect the dying patient—as well as protect the surgeon doing organ transplants from violating the law. But this was not the only reason to redefine death: "Of 36 comatose patients who were declared dead on the basis of irreversible loss of brain functions, only six were organ donors . . . thus, medical concern over the determination of death rests much less with any wish to facilitate organ transplantation than with the need both to render appropriate care to patients and to replace artificial support with more fitting and respectful behavior when a patient has become a dead body" (President's Commission, Note 1).

Robert Veatch, the noted medical ethicist, proposes four separate levels in order to arrive at a definition of death: first, "a complete change in the status of a living entity characterized by the irreversible loss of those characteristics that are essentially significant to it. It would be the point at which the individual is no longer treated as a human being." Second, there must be a concept of death. What is that part of life that when it is lost there is death? Is life defined by the flow of vital fluids, the breath, or blood; is life in the soul or in our capacity for bodily integration or in our capacity for social interaction?

Third, once we have defined our concept of death, we must determine its locus. If our concept of death concerns the loss of vital fluids, then we must look at the heart and lungs. If one is concerned with bodily integration, then one focuses on the total brain; if the concept is based on social interaction, then death would probably occur in the neocortex. For the soul, one might look to the pineal body, as was suggested by the philosopher Descartes.

Fourth, the criteria of death should be determined. What specific tests—an electroencephalogram, for example?—must be applied at the locus of death to see if death has occurred? The criteria used to measure death should stem from our concept of death. They should not be affected by our need for organs for transplantations, nor by economic considerations (Veatch, Note 2).

Today, legislation accepts either the brain or the heart and lungs as the locus of death. In the United States, the 1981 President's Commission for the Study of Ethical Problems in Medicare and Biomedical and Behavioral Research proposed a definition of death which would unify the various definitions proposed by different states: "An individual who has sustained either (1) irreversible cessation of circulatory and respiratory functions, or (2) irreversible cessation of all functions of the entire brain, including the brain stem, is dead. A determination of death must be made in accordance with accepted medical standards" (President's Commission, Note 3).

New Questions about Brain Death

With this definition of death, the question now arises as to whether death should be defined as the irreversible loss of consciousness, or the capacity for social interaction, which is located only in the higher brain, the part concerned with consciousness, speech, and feeling. The lower brain, the brain stem, which is responsible for respiration and spontaneous vegetative functions, also contributes to the maintenance of blood pressure. Although the lower brain can continue to function without the higher brain, the opposite cannot occur.

Changing the definition of death to include only loss of higher brain functions would affect two groups of people: those individuals who are in a persistent vegetative state, and babies who are born anencephalic, that is, with only a brain stem. Persons in a persistent vegetative state have a higher brain that no longer functions, yet they continue to breathe because of their brain stem. Such was the case with Karen Ann Quinlan. After the courts resolved that she could be removed from a respirator, she continued to breathe on her own. If the definition of death were different, she would have been considered dead. The fear about changing the definition of death is that persons in a persistent vegetative state could be misdiagnosed and could be defined as dead when there is a chance for recovery. There is also the "slippery slope" argument: that if the definition of death were to be changed, it could ultimately lead to declaring people dead who merely lack certain mental abilities.

Anencephalic babies only have a brain stem. They will continue to breath after birth. The question of whether they should be considered dead is especially important because of the viability of the babies' organs for transplants. Two cases illustrate the difficulties involved in declaring anencephalic babies to be dead. In 1987, parents of Baby Gabrielle knew that their baby would be born anencephalic, yet they decided that they wanted their infant's organs used for transplantation, to contribute to life in some way. The baby was kept on life supports and died 2 days after birth, when her heart was transplanted into Baby Paul. In 1992, parents of Baby Theresa Ann made a similar decision. However, they asked the Florida courts to declare Theresa Ann dead, although her heart was beating. The judges refused to do so, basing their decision on the fact that Baby Theresa Ann had brain stem activity, and therefore did not meet the requirements for the legal definition of death. The baby continued to breathe, but her organs deteriorated, and they were unable to be used for transplants.

Many ethicists believe that an exception to the brain death definition should be made in cases of anencephaly, since the higher brain is absent. The argument that a margin of safety must exist before a person is declared dead, as with someone in a persistent vegetative state, does not seem to hold here. As ethicist Robert Levine states, "With anencephalics you don't have to be extra safe. They never had sentient lives and never will" (Levine, Note 4). Yet, if the definition of death were to be changed to include only the higher brain, whether for those in a persistent vegetative state or for babies who are anencephalic, we would need to be declaring as dead those persons who are still breathing.

THE RIGHT TO REFUSE TREATMENT

The principle that adults have a right to refuse treatment was stated in 1914 by Judge Benjamin Cardozo: "Every human being of adult years and sound mind has a right to determine what shall be done with his own body; and a surgeon who performs an operation without his patient's consent commits an assault, for which he is liable in damages" (Cardozo, Note 5).

This right was reconfirmed by the U.S. Supreme Court in 1990 in the Nancy Cruzan case: "The principle that a competent person has a constitutionally protected liberty interest in refusing unwanted medical treatment may be inferred from our prior decisions," wrote Chief Justice Rehnquist in his opinion. The decision was based on the Fourteenth Amendment to the U.S. Constitution, which traces its roots to English common law, where "even the touching of one person by another without consent and without legal justification was a battery" (New York Times, Note 6). This led to the patient's right to informed consent, which means that the patient must be told of the risks involved in any treatment and that he or she must consent to the treatment. Implicit in the principle of informed consent is the principle of informed refusal.

The loophole in the right to refuse treatment is that the adult must be "competent." However, various groups have suggested that the capacity or capability to make a decision, rather than competency, should be the issue. The 1967 *Guidelines on the Termination of Life Sustaining Treatment and the Care of the Dying*, published by the Hastings Center, Hastings, New York, define decision-making capacity as (1) the ability to comprehend information relevant to the decision, (2) the ability to deliberate about the choices in accordance with personal values and goals, and (3) the ability to communicate (verbally or nonverbally) with caregivers.

If a person is capable of making a health care decision, then he or she should have the right to refuse treatment. But what if a person is not able to make such a decision? The following trends have emerged from court cases: "An adult patient's right to accept or refuse medical treatment continues even though he or she loses the capacity to make such a decision personally; a patient's incapacity to make a specific decision about medical treatment can differ from a judicial determination of a person's general incompetence; a nonautonomous patient's surrogate has the legal authority to accept or refuse medical treatment on behalf of the patient . . ." (Weir, Note 7).

This issue of the capacity to decide was central to the 1976 case of Joseph Saikewicz, a man who had developed acute myeloblastic monocytic leukemia, which is considered incurable. Chemotherapy is generally administered, however, in the hope that the therapy will be successful and the patient will go into remission. The treatment is painful, it has serious side effects, and it requires the patient's cooperation. Without the treatment, the patient will definitely die in a short time but will die painlessly. The difficulty with this case was that Mr. Saikewicz was a severely retarded, institutionalized 67-year-old man. The guardian appointed for Mr. Saikewicz eventually recommended that he not be given chemotherapy. This was accepted by the probate court, but the judge also referred the case for review. The Supreme Court of Massachusetts approved the lower court's decision, issuing a full opinion in November 1977; meanwhile, Mr. Saikewicz had died in September 1976. The decision to withhold treatment in this case was not based on Mr. Saikewicz's incompetency. Rather, the court reaffirmed "that the noncompetent person has the same rights with respect to care as the competent person." The reason that treatment was withheld was that it would have led to a great deal of pain and disorientation for Mr. Saikewicz.

Advance Directives

One way to address the issue of patients making their own health care decisions is to have them make out documents while they are capable of making decisions, to prepare for if and when they are not capable of making decisions. There are two types of such advance directives: a treatment directive or "living will," and a proxy directive allowing a surrogate to make treatment decisions.

A living will is a document that allows a person to specify what treatment, if any, he or she would want to be given under certain conditions. Although now enforceable in most states, only a small proportion of patients have made out living wills. One problem with living wills is that they are usually couched in general terms, so that a surrogate is needed to interpret the patient's intentions.

A proxy directive is an advance directive whereby an individual appoints someone else to make health care decisions if he or she becomes incapable of doing so. This could take the form of a durable power of attorney.

Children and the Refusal of Treatment

When the patient is a minor, it is the parents who must authorize treatment. If physicians (or others) disagree with the parents' decision, it becomes subject to judicial review. Where the child is not in danger of dying, the courts have decided based on the reasonableness of the parents' decision. There are generally three acceptable reasons for refusing treatment: when the treatment carries substantial risk; when there is no clear need for treatment; and when the treatment can be delayed until the child can be consulted.

If a dying child can be restored to health through medical treatment that the parents refuse, the courts will intervene. For example, blood transfusions have been ordered for children of Jehovah's Witnesses, because the courts have decided that there is no parental right to allow their children to die needlessly.

In 1984, Congress amended the Child Abuse and Neglect Prevention and Treatment Act to define withholding of treatment from an infant as a form of child abuse, except in three cases: "for infants who are irreversibly comatose; for infants for whom such treatment would prolong dying; or for infants for whom such treatment would be 'virtually futile' and its provision would be inhumane." Hence, babies born with defects, who are not terminally ill, would be treated. This amendment came about as a result of two cases.

Baby Doe of Indiana was born in 1982 with Down's syndrome and a gastrointestinal malformation. The parents decided against surgery. The hospital contested the parents' decision, arguing that the malformation was surgically correctable. The Indiana Supreme Court upheld the parents' decision. Baby Doe died 6 days later.

On October 11, 1983, Baby Jane Doe of New York was born with spina bifida, hydrocephalus (water on the brain), and other disorders. The parents refused surgery that might have extended the child's life from 2 to 20 years. New York's highest court upheld the parents' decision, declaring that it was "well within medical standards and there was no medical reason to disturb the parents' decision." Certainly, the child was in no immediate danger.

Under the new regulations, Baby Doe of Indiana would have probably had the surgery; it is not clear what would have happened to Baby Jane Doe. One result of the new regulations is that hospitals are now taking a "treat, wait, and see" approach to the care of newborns. Assessments concerning further care are then made and the decisions revolve around withdrawing treatment rather than withholding it.

EUTHANASIA

Euthanasia, which comes from the Greek words for "good death," has come to encompass four different ethical policies: making the terminal stages of illness as painless as possible, but not hastening death; making the terminal stage as painless as possible, and condoning jeopardizing the patient's life in the process; ceasing or not starting treatment; and actively participating in ending the patient's life (Reiser, Note 8). Euthanasia may be applied to persons with terminal disease, persons in irreversible comas, or persons, although not terminally ill, whose quality of life is unacceptable.

In discussions of euthanasia, major distinctions must be made between active and passive euthanasia; direct and indirect euthanasia; and voluntary and involuntary euthanasia.

Active and Passive

The major difference between active and passive, or positive and negative euthanasia, is that active euthanasia involves committing an act that would result in a person's death, whereas passive euthanasia involves omission of an act that would prolong life. Some ethicists see differences between active and passive euthanasia. First, the cause of death is different: In omission, the cause of death is the disease, not the action of another. Second, the long-range effects on society may be different. There is a possibility that if we allow active killing of those who are dying, we may consequently allow active killing of others. This "wedge argument" was used in Nazi Germany. As Leo Alexander, a physician who helped draft the Nuremberg Code, stated: "The German mass murders started with the acceptance of that attitude basic in the euthanasia movement, that there is such a thing as life not worthy to be lived. This attitude in its early stages concerned itself merely with the severely and chronically sick. Gradually, the sphere of those to be included was enlarged to include the socially unproductive, the racially unwanted, and finally all non-Germans. But it is important to realize that the infinitely small wedged-in lever from which the entire trend of mind received its impetus was the attitude toward the nonrehabilitable sick" (Veatch, Note 9). Third, while letting someone die may be fulfilling the principle of respecting their autonomy, killing is always a violation of the duty to avoid killing.

The law does make distinctions between active and passive euthanasia. Legally, active euthanasia is absolutely prohibited, since motive is no defense for killing. Those doctors and laypersons who have committed "mercy killings" have been acquitted on the basis of temporary insanity.

Today, a form of active euthanasia, assisted suicide, has become an important issue. The book *Final Exit* by Derek Humphrey (1990), is a best-selling suicide manual designed for the terminally ill that provides information on methods of committing suicide. A retired physician, Jack Kevorkian, has been in the news because he developed a "suicide machine" that allows a patient to give him or herself an intravenous injection of poison. Kevorkian's machine has been used by some nonterminally ill patients, such as Janet Adkins, who suffered from Alzheimer's disease. In the state of Washington, a 1991 referendum to legalize assisted suicide was voted down by 54% of the voters. The initiative would have allowed doctors to assist in suicide in cases where the patient was conscious and competent, the patient made a written request to die witnessed by two people, and two physicians had certified that the patient had less than six months to live. Measures of this type will probably appear on the ballot in other states.

Direct and Indirect

Direct and indirect forms of euthanasia are similar to passive and active forms. The distinction between direct and indirect killing lies in whether or not death is the primary intention of the act. The major indirect form of euthanasia is the use of painkilling drugs. To lessen the suffering of the patient, greater and greater dosages of a painkiller may be administered. Through doing this, death may be hastened, but since the primary intention in giving the medication was to lessen pain, the death would be indirect.

Voluntary and Involuntary

Voluntary euthanasia refers to euthanasia with patient consent, while involuntary euthanasia does not involve the patient's consent. The arguments against voluntary euthanasia are that the patient may not be making a decision based on personal wishes, but may be consenting to relieve the suffering of another, such as a family caregiver; that the patient may be in the midst of a temporary depression when deciding; and that medication may induce confusion, so that the person is actually unable to make a decision. The problem with voluntary euthanasia, of course, is that it is irreversible. Once the decision has been made and the treatment stopped, one cannot change one's mind. Proponents of voluntary euthanasia believe, nevertheless, that a person has the right to decide whether or not to continue living, and that safeguards, such as requiring a period of time between the request for euthanasia and the act itself, should be used to protect the patient.

Legal Issues of Euthanasia

Over the past 20 years the legal issues surrounding euthanasia have changed dramatically. There are basically six different positions held on euthanasia:

1. Life-sustaining treatment should never be withheld or stopped.

2. Treatment of nondying patients should never be withheld or stopped.

3. Life-sustaining nutrition and hydration should never be withheld or stopped.

4. All life-sustaining medical treatment should be withheld or stopped when warranted.

5. Intentional killing is acceptable as an exceptional moral alternative.

6. Intentional killing is acceptable as both a moral and a legal alternative (Weir, Note 10).

Although there are ethicists who take each of these six different positions, only positions 1 through 4 are now legal in the United States today.

Three significant years, 1976, 1985, and 1990, had events which led to major changes in the legal status of euthanasia. In 1976, Karen Ann Quinlan, a 21-year-old woman in a coma, was admitted to St. Clare's Hospital in Denville, New Jersey, where she was placed on a respirator. Several months later, her father signed a release permitting the physicians to turn off the respirator, which the physicians refused to do, stating that it would be an act of homicide. Karen Ann's father then went to court to be appointed her guardian, specifically to be granted "the express power of withdrawing treatment from Karen Ann," arguing that she would have wanted to be removed from the machine. The Superior Court, however, decided in favor of the hospital, claiming that Karen Ann Quinlan was still alive, that she did not meet the criteria for brain death, and that "there is a duty to continue the life assisting apparatus, if within the treating physician's opinion it should be done. . . . There is no constitutional right to die that can be asserted by a parent for his incompetent adult child." On appeal, the New Jersey Supreme Court overturned the lower court's ruling, partly based on the violation of Karen's right to privacy. The Supreme Court decided that if there were no reasonable possibility of Karen's ever becoming conscious, the life-support systems could be removed without any civil or criminal liability. Karen Ann Quinlan was then weaned from the respirator.

The second influence on the issue of euthanasia in 1976 was the formulation of Massachusetts General Hospital's do-not-resuscitate (DNR) regulations, which distinguished different levels of treatment for four different classes of patients. Class A patients were to receive maximal therapeutic effort without reservation. Class B and C patients were to receive more selective treatment, and for Class D patients, those with brain death or those with no chance of regaining "cognitive and sapient life," treatment would be discontinued.

The third event in 1976 was the passage of the California Natural Death Act, whereby California became the first state to recognize the legality of a living will. This document allowed a person to specify what treatment, if any, he or she would want, given a terminal condition.

In 1985, there were two more major developments. The New Jersey Supreme Court decided that a nasogastric tube, which provided artificial nutrition and hydration, could be removed from incompetent 83-year-old Claire Conroy at the behest of her legal guardian. The decision was based on an individual's "right to reject *any* medical treatment under the doctrine of informed consent." And, following California, 13 other states passed natural death acts in 1985 that contained language on nutrition and hydration. This brought the total of natural death acts to 36 (in 35 states and the District of Columbia). Hence, artificial hydration and nutrition could be treated as any other form of medical treatment, and refusal could be included in one's living will. This view of artificial hydration and nutrition was affirmed by the U.S. Supreme Court in 1990 with the Nancy Cruzan case.

In 1983, Nancy Cruzan had been in a car accident that left her in a persisten vegetative state; she could breathe but had no consciousness. Her life was maintained through artificial hydration and nutrition. She had left no written instructions concerning her wishes if she were to be in a comatose state. The Missouri Supreme Court upheld the Missouri law requiring "clear and convincing evidence" that a person would want treatment to be discontinued, and denied Cruzan's parents' request to remove the nasogastric tube. On June 25, 1990, however, the U.S. Supreme Court, while upholding Missouri's and all states' rights to require such evidence, ended the distinction between artificial feeding and other medical treatment. The

Court also acknowledged that competent persons have a constitutional right to refuse medical treatment.

Religious Issues of Euthanasia

Religion plays an important role in the issue of euthanasia. The views of Catholicism, Orthodox Judaism, and Fundamentalist Protestantism are opposed to any form of active euthanasia, but there are allowances made for forms of passive euthanasia.

The Catholic view of euthanasia, reaffirmed in 1984 by the National Conference of Catholic Bishops, was first stated by Pope Pius XII in 1957 in his *allocutio* to Italian anesthetists. Accordingly, direct euthanasia is strictly forbidden; if self-administered, it is suicide, and if death is administered by another, it is homicide. Passive euthanasia is limited by the distinction between ordinary and extraordinary procedures. Ordinary measures must always be applied; otherwise, it is morally the same as killing the patient. The exclusion of extraordinary treatments where there is no reasonable hope of recovery is acceptable. However, doctors and moralists use the terms *ordinary* and *extraordinary* in different ways. The physician is likely to define ordinary as standard, well-established, customary procedures, without taking into account the medical history of the patient. The moralist might define ordinary as any measure, experimental or unorthodox, that could reasonably help the patient.

Judaism, too, does not sanction active euthanasia, finding a biblical basis for the view in the words of King David, who refused to allow the badly wounded King Saul to be killed in order to relieve his suffering. In terms of passive euthanasia, however, the degree of acceptance is related to the orthodoxy of the theologian. The Orthodox Jewish tradition sanctions the withdrawal of any factor that may artificially delay the patient's death in the *final phase*, a period of three days or less. Conservative and Reform Jews would define passive euthanasia with fewer limitations on the prognosis of the dying individual.

Protestantism provides very different views on euthanasia. Karl Barth, a prominent Swiss Protestant theologian, believes that human life belongs solely to God, and that we are wrongfully killing a person when we allow him or her to die. At the other end of the debate, however, is the Protestant view that defines euthanasia as merciful release from incurable suffering, a decision that depends on the situation of the dying person. Different Protestant denominations reflect different views. Southern Baptists, for example, are opposed to all forms of euthanasia, while the United Church of

Christ passed a resolution affirming "individual freedom and responsibility" in making choices around euthanasia and suicide.

REFERENCE NOTES

1. President's Commission for the Study of Ethical Problems in Medical and Biomedical and Behavioral Research. *Defining death*. Washington, D.C.: U.S. Government Printing Office, 1981, pp. 23–24.
2. Veatch, R., *Death, dying and the biological revolution* (rev. ed.). New Haven, Ct.: Yale University Press, 1989.
3. President's Commission, op. cit., p. 2.
4. Levine, R., as quoted in Chartrand, S. Baby missing part of brain challenges legal definition of death. *New York Times*. March 29, 1992, p. 12.
5. Cardozo, B., as quoted in Grisez, G. & Boyle, J. *Life and death with liberty and justice*. Notre Dame, Ind.: University of Notre Dame Press, 1979, p. 88.
6. *New York Times*, June 26, 1990, A1 and A19.
7. Weir, R. *Abating treatment with critically ill patients*. New York: Oxford University Press, 1989, p. 145.
8. Reiser, S. The dilemma of euthanasia in modern medical history: The english and american experience. In J. Behake and S. Bok (eds.), *The dilemmas of euthanasia*. Garden City, N.Y.: Schor Press, 1975, p. 31.
9. Veatch, R. op. cit., p. 66.
10. Weir, R. op. cit., pp. 227–268.

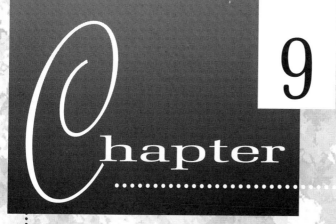

Chapter 9

Suicide

While suicide has existed throughout civilization, attitudes toward it have fluctuated, largely depending on the time in history and how a particular culture views death. In ancient Greece, suicide was accepted by many philosophers as a reasonable choice, and throughout Japanese history suicide has been an expression of various aspects of personal honor.

According to early Christianity, suicide was regarded as a mortal sin and a serious offense against society and the state. Until the end of the eighteenth century, people in France who attempted suicide and failed were sometimes hanged. If they succeeded in killing themselves, their bodies were sometimes dragged through the streets or thrown onto the public garbage dump. When people committed suicide in England during the eighteenth century, their estate could be turned over to the crown, and often they were buried at a crossroads with a stake through their heart.

Attitudes toward suicide arising from the Age of Enlightenment were more humanistic. Early nineteenth century Romantics considered suicide to be rather heroic and poetic. In the twentieth century, suicide in the Western world has come to be viewed more in medical and psychological terms. Factors that may influence the attitudes of people toward suicide and suicidal behaviors include age, sex, race, and education level. In a study of college students' attitudes toward suicide, it was found that evaluation of suicide tended to be more favorable when the evaluators were male, when male victims were being judged, when elderly victims were being evaluated, and when terminal cancer was the precipitating factor. Yet despite vast amounts of literature and discussion about death by suicide, it still remains an enigma.

WHO ATTEMPTS OR COMMITS SUICIDE?

According to data tabulated by the National Center for Health Statistics in 1991, the suicide rate in the United States was 11.4 per 100,000 persons. In 1990, suicide ranked as one of the ten leading causes of death. Demographic risk factors often associated with suicide include age, sex, race, marital status, affective disorders, alcoholism, lack of social support, history of previous suicidal attempts, and mental illness, although some of these factors are controversial.

The accuracy of statistics about suicide is often questioned. There is still some social stigma attached to suicide, especially with children, which may lead to an underreporting and a covering up of suicidal behavior. Suicides may also be underreported since many deaths that are designated as accidents, such as one-car automobile accidents and drownings, may actually have been suicides. Statistics can, however, provide some basic information about the epidemiology of suicide. With this in mind, key demographic considerations of age, race, and gender as they relate to suicide are explored further here.

Age

Data from the Centers for Disease Control (1986) and the National Center for Health Statistics (1988) indicate that suicide rates for adolescents 15 to 19 years of age had quadrupled in the preceding 40 years. The reasons for this are multiple and complex. Adolescence is a tumultuous time that marks the transition into adulthood; the fragmentation of family life, shifts in cultural mores, pressures of parents with high expectations, and problems with interpersonal relationships are further contributing factors for teenagers. An important predictor of adolescent suicide is the occurrence and seriousness of a previous attempt. Other known risk factors include social isolation, depression, alcohol and other drug use, and access to lethal means of committing suicide. Homosexuality is also a risk factor. One researcher has noted that most suicide attempts by homosexuals occur during their youth, and gay youths appear to be two or three times more likely to attempt suicide than other young people (Gibson, Note 1).

The increase in suicide within the adolescent age group has been greatest among young white men, with an increase being noted each year for the past 25 years. Suicide rates for African American youths in this age group have also increased, and rates for young black men are over four times the rate for young women.

At the other end of the age spectrum, the elderly have a rate of suicide that is more than double that in the general population. Currently, elderly white men are the most vulnerable group for suicide in people age 65 and older. African Americans and Native Americans have a decrease in suicide rates after age 40. One reason for this lower incidence of nonwhite elderly suicide may be the extension of traditional values of respect for the elderly in nonwhite cultures that give the elderly members a sense of dignity and worth that keeps them from feeling suicidal (Nkongho, Note 2).

There are a number of explanations for the generally high elderly suicide rate in the United States, some of which are based on the intense and accelerated rate of change people experience as they age. These changes include significant life events such as retirement, loss of a spouse, shrinking income, deteriorating health, and loss of friends. It is also important to consider how elderly people are valued in American society. Many view the elderly as no longer contributing to production and therefore see them as a burden and a drain on the tax base, as they require Social Security and health care benefits. Some elderly people may internalize such perceptions and experience a loss of self-esteem and meaning in their life, which can lead to depression and the ultimate response of suicide.

Race and Culture

Recent data on African American suicide rates show them to be lower across all age groups and both genders than those of whites, with the brunt of African American suicide being borne by the 25- to 34-year-old age group. While many factors in suicidal behavior—anger, low self-esteem, depression, an inability to express feelings, and difficulties in family structure—are present among all groups, some researchers believe that a sociological frame of reference is critical to examining suicide among African Americans, and that issues such as racism, oppression, poor education, and unemployment are central.

In addition to the sociological perspective, some researchers have used a psychosocial framework to theorize about suicide among African Americans. One study of young suicidal African Americans in a ghetto environment, for example, indicates that the young people feel trapped at an early age in an unalterable life situation: trapped by lack of education and job opportunities, and by the destructive effects of the ghetto on their own personalities. While such studies may be illuminating, more research is needed to identify the strengths in the African American community that have kept the suicide rate lower than that of the white community.

There are few publications in the literature on suicidal behavior among Latinos. In looking at this issue, it is important to remember that the Latino population is not homogeneous; characteristics of the various subgroups may be different. Research seems to indicate that Latino suicides are primarily young men, but across all age groups Latinos appear half as likely as whites to commit suicide. Perhaps the lower Latino suicide rates may be attributed to the influence of such values as family honor, solidarity, and kinship support.

Among Native American peoples, there are tremendous variations in social, economic, and educational factors, which result in a diversity of behavior regarding suicide. Perhaps since Native American suicide rates often fluctuate with those of their surrounding communities, these rates should be compared to those of neighboring general populations. In general, emerging characteristics of Native American suicide appear to include the following: suicide is predominantly carried out by men age 15 to 24; groups with loose social integration and a high degree of individuality appear to have higher suicide rates than those with tight integration, which emphasizes conformity; groups undergoing rapid social and economic changes have higher suicide rates than those who are not. Loss of traditional culture and loss of control over one's life may be other important factors, although there have been few scientific studies into the relevance of these and other factors in suicide among Native Americans.

As with the term *Latino*, Asian American covers a wide range of people from many countries, with diverse languages and cultures. Asian Americans include Chinese, Japanese, Koreans, Filipinos, Southeast Asians, Indians, Pakistanis, Sri Lankans, and Pacific Islanders. The most consistent and reliable data on suicide among Asian American groups in the United States are those relating to Chinese and Japanese Americans.

Historically, as noted earlier, suicide in Japan has met with religious tolerance and state approval, and Japan has a higher suicide rate than the United States. In the United States, however, Japanese Americans have a generally lower suicide rate that that of white Americans. There is a minor peak in suicide rates among young adult Japanese Americans and a major peak among the elderly.

In contrast with the Japanese, the Chinese have no tradition of suicide as a socially acceptable response to difficult circumstances. Suicide rates among Chinese Americans are generally lower than those for white Americans. However, the rates are similarly distributed by age, with peak rates among those age 65 and older. There is a high incidence of suicide among older Chinese American women as compared with men, which is different from the rates among elderly white Americans.

The process of acculturation is relevant to the phenomenon of suicide among Asian Americans. The language barrier can be a major problem for Asian immigrants. In addition, there is sometimes a lack of community resources to help Asian immigrants with adaptation and acculturation. This is true, for example, for Chinese immigrants. In the case of suicidal behavior, there is a need for caregivers who understand Asian cultural differences to participate in treatment of Asian immigrants. Being able to give more concrete and directive advice would be useful, for example, and involving family members in psychotherapy when treating the suicidal Asian patient is of particular importance.

Gender

In the general population, one of the most evident conclusions about suicide is that men commit suicide at a rate two to three times higher than women. Women, on the other hand, *attempt* suicide three to five times more than men. It may be that men are more often completers of suicide than women due to differences in the methods employed by the two sexes. Statistical reports of the highly lethal use of firearms by more male suicides than female suicides cannot be understood without reference to the cultural context in which the suicide occurs. No one would be surprised to learn that women have had less access to lethal weapons than men. The method of suicide thus must be considered not only in terms of gender but also in relation to cultural and to psychosocial factors.

So long as the study of suicide and suicidal behavior continues to focus on completed suicide, it will remain a study of a male issue and will exclude the cultural, social, and personal factors to be found in women's experiences. Not only is attempted suicide a more common behavior, it may also be more rational and adaptive. It is important that both attempted and completed suicide be studied so the findings will encompass the reality of suicide for both women and men.

Thus, among the many variables which may influence the phenomenon of suicide are age, race, culture, gender, religious beliefs, socioeconomic stress, alcohol and other drug use, and affective disorders. A number of theories have been developed to explain suicide.

THEORIES OF SUICIDE

No one really knows why people kill themselves. Attempts to examine and explain the etiology of suicide have been many and varied and have included ethical, familial, interpersonal, and political approaches. Those discussed here fall into the categories of (1) philosophical, (2) sociological, (3) psychoanalytical, (4) biochemical, and (5) preventionist theories.

Philosophical

Philosophers have not provided one specific theory of suicide. The philosophy of existentialism as articulated by the French philosopher Albert Camus identifies suicide as the only serious philosophical question. If life is absurd and meaningless, as existentialism suggests, then death is also absurd. Therefore, according to Camus, the individual should resist the temptation of suicide and somehow continue to live in this "absurd state," constantly confronting the world. It is confrontation that gives life meaning. Other philosophers disagree, however, and state viewpoints that are more permissive of suicide.

Sociological

Some theories of suicide take into consideration the cultural context of the individual and how the individual relates to that context. These models lay varying emphasis on the individual's adjustment to the social order and the strength of that social order's ability to influence suicide.

The classic study of suicide in the context of the social order was done by the nineteenth century French sociologist Émile Durkheim. He proposed that to understand suicide rates, it was necessary to examine social forces rather than isolated individual motives. A major component of Durkheim's thesis was the capacity of the individual to be adequately integrated into the prevailing social structures, such as religion, family, and community. The more an individual was integrated, the less the likelihood of suicide.

Durkheim categorized suicide into three types according to its social context: "egoistic" suicide, the suicide of the poorly integrated individual; "altruistic" suicide, the suicide of the individual who is willing, even eager, to sacrifice his or her life to a social cause; and "anomic" suicide, which occurs when a person experiences a sense of anomy and alienation, often because society is changing rapidly and there are no new rules to take the place of the old ones that are breaking down. Personal changes such as divorce, and socioeconomic changes such as the Great Depression of the 1930s may be precipitating crises for anomic suicide.

An additional category, egocentric suicide, has been suggested as one that places a greater emphasis on frustration and aggression in contrast to the loss and despair of egoistic suicide. While Durkheim's theory has been useful in examining causes of suicide and suicide rates, it cannot be used to understand an individual's psychological motivation for suicide. While all three categories revolve around a person's integration into society, the theory cannot explain why some people who are single, widowed, or divorced kill themselves, when most do not (Colt, Note 3).

Psychoanalytical

In 1910, 13 years after Durkheim published his theory of suicide, suicide was the topic at the Vienna Psychoanalytic Society. At that time, Sigmund Freud cautioned that suicide was still an unresolved problem, and he continued to question self-destructive behavior. His classic paper, "Mourning and Melancholia," published in 1917, dealt with the dynamics of depression. Freud formulated the view that suicide is a form of aggression against an internalized love object. Since the person both loves and hates at the same time, this aggression is markedly ambivalent.

Karl Menninger elaborated on Freud's theory of aggression turned inward (Menninger, Note 4). He believed that any suicide is driven by three conscious or unconscious wishes: the wish to kill, the wish to be killed, and the wish to die. Currently, additional emphasis is placed on the importance of the feelings of helplessness, hopelessness, and dependency in self-destructive behavior. These feelings, when severe, are characteristics of depression and severely depressed individuals are at risk for suicide.

The psychoanalytic approach, which proposes that changes in instinctual drives and unconscious motivation give rise to suicidal behavior, is the most obvious choice to illustrate individual-oriented approaches to suicide, and much of contemporary nursing, psychiatry, psychology, and social work have benefited from the early work of Freud and other psychoanalysts. However, it has also been evident for several decades that a truly psychosocial approach, which incoporates the work of Freud and Durkheim but also examines the psychodynamics of suicide in different social groups, is required for any deeper understanding of suicide in a particular society. Psychic, social, cultural, and physiological factors all interact to produce self-destructive behavior.

Biochemical

Historically, in an attempt to understand suicide, physicians searched for its cause within the body itself. In doing so, a medical model for suicide as a disease was formed, separating it from suicide as a moral problem. Suicide was attributed to climate, change of season, heredity, insanity, constipation, and numerous other causes, depending on the diagnosing physician. One early nineteenth century physician wrote that suicide was not a disease per se but a symptom, and that the treatment of suicide belonged to the therapy of mental illness. The psychiatric theory of suicide today makes a similar assumption, that most people who kill themselves suffer from a mental or emotional disorder.

Current research in the physiological study of suicide indicates promising findings in the biochemical area. There is developing evidence that suicidal behaviors may be associated with abnormalities in the serotonergic system. Serotonin is a neurotransmitter that carries chemical messages between neurons in the brain, affecting how people feel and think. Numerous reports indicate that low levels of a serotonin metabolite (a breakdown product of serotonin) called 5-hydroxyindoleacetic acid (5-HIAA) have been found in the cerebrospinal fluid of suicidal patients with psychiatric diagnoses, including depressive illness, personality disorder, schizophrenia, and alcoholism (Stanley and Stanley, Note 5).

Moreover, one recent report shows that self-destructive behavior is associated with disturbances in serotonin turnover: in completed suicides, studies of brain regions and cerebrospinal fluid indicate a dysfunction of the serotonergic system. There has also been some evidence of certain endocrine functions, particularly the release of cortisol and thyrotropin, associated with suicidal behavior.

Clearly much more research needs to be done to determine more exact relationships between low serotonin and suicidal behavior. However, it is possible that behavioral markers of suicide may be combined with biological markers to predict suicide for certain populations of patients. Such a possibility holds great promise for prevention.

Preventionist

The Suicide Prevenion Center in Los Angeles, established in 1958, was a pioneering agency in the analysis of suicide from a prevention perspective. Research done at the center concluded that the majority of suicides have a recognizable presuicidal phase. In reconstructing events preceding a death by means of a psychological autopsy, to help answer questions of why, how, and what, the center concluded that suicidal behavior is often a form of communication, a call for help. Preventionist theory recognizes in these calls for help the potential for intervention in suicidal behavior.

Edwin Shneidman, a prominent researcher in suicide behavior, suggests that any suicide is colored with ambivalence: He has various categories of death-related behavior that include intentioned, unintentioned, and subintentioned death (Shneidman, Note 6). In intentioned death, the individual takes a direct, active role in bringing about death. The "death-seeker" may commit suicide "in such a manner that rescue is realistically unlikely or impossible"; the "death-initiator" believes death will occur soon and precipitates the event. An example of a death-initiator would be an older person in the terminal stage of a fatal illness who commits suicide. A third kind of intentioned death would be that of the "death-ignorer," who believes that life will continue in some other fashion. A final category is the "death-darer," the person who tempts fate by engaging in risky methods, such as Russian roulette.

Unintentioned death occurs when the individual plays no significant role in precipitating death. Different attitudes are attributed in unintentioned death, however. The "death welcomer" is glad that death will occur; the "death-acceptor" is resigned to his or her fate; the "death-postponer" endeavors to forestall death; the "death-disdainer" does not believe death will occur; and the "death-fearer" is fearful and fights the notion of death.

Shneidman also accounts for suicide by subintentional death, when the person plays a partial or unconscious role in hastening his or her own death. In subintentional death, the individual unconsciously allows suicide to occur through his or her behavior. The "death-darer" and the "death-chancer" play a game to court death with odds calculated in their favor. The "death-hastener" unconsciously brings about or exacerbates a physiological imbalance.

The individual who has a destructive life-style, such as through alcohol, drug, or dietary abuse, or who refuses to follow medical orders for a specific condition, is considered to be a death-hastener. A "death-facilitator" will passively make death easy. The "death-capitulator" plays a psychological role, usually through fear, in terminating life. Voodoo deaths fall into this category. Finally, the "death-experimenter" lives on the brink of death, usually by excessive use of alcohol or drugs that bring about an altered, usually befogged, state of consciousness.

Furthermore, there is also suicide by murder, when an individual purposely chooses a superior adversary and thus brings about his or her own death. This "victim-precipitated" homicide is another form of subintentional death. An example of this would be when a person brandishes a gun, knowing it is unloaded, in front of police officers, provoking them to shoot in apparent self-defense. However, this type of situation must be interpreted carefully to avoid blaming the victim for the brutal acts of another. The issues regarding subintentional deaths for health care professionals and for society at large are multiple. Should these deaths be accepted as suicides? Are they preventable? What mode of intervention would be most effective?

Some suicide analysts have criticized the preceding theoretical approaches to suicide, because these theories tend to separate suicidal individuals from the context of their experience. Suicide theories must take into account the multiple variables influencing the suicidal person and consider the increasing social isolation that occurs as the suicidal individual experiences hopelessness, helplessness, and failure.

In the meantime, as analysts consider suicide from various perspectives, the suicidal crisis requires immediate action. The health care practitioner feels compelled to act; the life that is saved today is the life that matters. And indeed, while suicide is an enormously complicated problem, "it is not totally random and it is amenable to some prediction . . . and to effective therapeutic intervention: that is reason for prevention" (Shneidman, Note 7).

SUICIDE PREVENTION

Prior to the 1950s and the advent of the Los Angeles Suicide Prevention Center, *suicide* was still a taboo word, and little attention was focused on it as a problem that needed to be treated. Concern over suicide became more highly formalized in the 1960s with the National Institute of Mental Health's establishment of a national coordinating effort on suicide prevention, and suicide prevention centers and suicide hot lines developed throughout the United States.

Suicide prevention centers, many of which now call themselves crisis intervention centers to reach a greater number of high-risk callers, came under close scrunity in the 1970s as to their effectiveness in actually preventing suicide. Some research indicated that suicide prevention centers do not affect community suicide rates. Additionally, some people question the ethics involved in suicide prevention, believing that people have a right to take their own life. However, the continued existence of suicide prevention–crisis intervention centers does indicate that they are meeting some community needs. Results of a study comparing suicide rates in counties that added these prevention centers between 1968 and 1973 with counties that did not indicated that the centers were associated with a reduction of suicides among young white women.

Calls for help to crisis intervention hot lines involve not only suicide but also rape, wife battering, child abuse, elder abuse, HIV and AIDS, substance abuse, and homelessness. The effectiveness of the centers may need to be evaluated in terms other than the decrease of suicide rates in the community. The establishment of a caring connection between the high-risk caller and the person answering the phone at the center help deter the caller from carrying out destructive behavior toward him or herself or toward others. As society in the United States becomes increasingly pluralistic, crisis centers will need to plan for intervention in a variety of modes. People of color will make up one-third of the population by the year 2000. Cultures differ widely with regard to their attitudes toward suicidal behavior and to the acceptability of programs that speak openly and frankly about it. To have even a modest chance of enduring success, prevention programs must be oriented to family, school, workplace, and larger community contexts as well as to the individual.

Assessing Suicidal Behavior

To assess whether an individual is thinking about committing suicide, it is important to dispel a number of common myths surrounding the subject. First, it is a myth that people who talk about suicide will not commit suicide. Suicide threats and warnings must be taken very seriously. Being alert to clues and indications of an intent to commit suicide is important. Furthermore, once the suicidal crisis passes, it is a myth that the risk is over. In fact, most suicides occur within 90 days of the initial emotional crisis, as the person appears to have recovered. This is a period in which physicians, relatives, and others should be especially watchful.

Second, while suicide and depression are not synonymous, depression does remain the best indicator of potential suicide. The majority of people who commit suicide are unhappy, temporarily overwhelmed individuals. It is not useful to consider suicide from the point of view of morality or criminality; it is a harmful myth that moral arguments or legislation will prevent suicide. In fact, they may do the opposite by preventing suicidal individuals from trying to seek help.

Many people falsely believe that suicide is inherited, but in fact it does not run in families. Furthermore, suicide cuts across all strata of society, rich and poor. Most important, it is dangerous to think that suicidal people are fully committed to dying and that suicide cannot be prevented. Most suicidal people are ambivalent about dying and can be saved and helped through proper assessment of distress signals and therapeutic intervention.

Prodromal indicators—signals of suicidal intentions, the cues, the "cries for help"—include the following:

- Verbal communication, such as statements that the person wishes he or she were dead, that the family would be better off without him or her.
- A history of suicide attempts.
- Unexplained changes in behavior, such as giving away important personal possessions, taking daredevil chances, becoming a reckless driver, irregular work attendance.
- Depression symptoms, including loss of appetite, weight loss, early waking, loss of energy, loss of interest in usual pleasures, social withdrawal, and severe feelings of hopelessness and helplessness.
- Physical illness. An estimated 75% of all suicides see a doctor in the 4 months before they take their life. A suicidal person may be using physical complaints as a way of seeking help from a physician. Physicians should take the time to explore how the person is feeling when no physical basis can be found for the chief complaint. People who are experiencing a disabling illness or one that is unresponsive to treatment can be considered at risk for suicide, as can people who

receive a diagnosis of an illness that may be life-threatening, such as cancer or HIV infection.

- A recent loss, such as the death of a loved one; divorce or separation; loss of a job, money, prestige, or status; loss of health; forced retirement.
- Drinking and other substance abuse. Alcohol and other drugs can increase impulsive behavior and impair judgment. Agencies and individuals involved in treating alcoholics and substance abusers should be alert to the risk of suicide among their clients and should be trained to identify and deal with an increased risk of suicidal behavior.

Assessment and Intervention

People may exhibit one or more of the prodromal indicators listed and not be suicidal, but if these prodromal indicators are present, it is important to assess and evaluate the individual's potential for suicide. It may be helpful to engage the person in a series of escalating questions that can create a more meaningful interaction and may help to overcome some of the person's resistance. In an assessment interview, it is important for caregivers to convey a real caring and concern for the person's distress as well as an acknowledgment of that person's strengths.

The following data need to be included and evaluated in an assessment of suicidal behavior:

- Suicide plan. Include queries about lethality of method, availability of method, and the specific organization of a suicide plan, including time and place.
- Severity of symptoms. Assess the level of distress: severe agitation, a sense of helplessness combined with a frantic need to do something, hopelessness that worsens when offered help. Is there psychotic thinking ("the voices are telling me to hurt myself")?
- Resources and communication. Does the person have any available support systems—family, friends, agencies, employer, therapists? What is and has been the extent of communication with these support systems? Are they available to help? Is the person financially stable?
- Precipitating stress. Stress should be evaluated from the person's standpoint, because people can perceive the meaning, degree, and intensity of stress quite differently. For example, the loss of a pet, which may have been an elderly person's only love object, may be

devastating to that person. Determine if the time of crisis coincides with a special anniversary date of a significant event in the person's life.

- Reaction of a significant other. Is the person supportive: does he or she show feelings of concern or recognize the need for help?

Suicide intervention can be primary, secondary, and tertiary. In the primary stage, the assessment is made and appropriate action is taken. If lethality of the situation is low, support from family, friends, and others may be sufficient. A highly lethal suicidal crisis requires referral to a mental health practitioner, mental health center, or crisis center. During the primary stage it is particularly important that the potentially suicidal person is "heard." Caregivers should be aware of the prodromal clues of suicide and feel comfortable enough to question the patient. It is not true that talking about suicide with people who are upset may encourage them to attempt suicide. In fact, suicide is much too complex to be caused simply by a caring person asking a question about suicidal intent. After an evaluation has been made, the caregiver should continue to be available to supply direct support and to assist the suicidal individual in following through on appropriate recommendations.

In caring for a dying patient, statements such as "I can't go on" or "I wish this were over" and actions such as writing a will are more commonplace. They should not be overlooked, however, as possible prodromal clues to suicide. Caregivers should take the time to explore the intent of the communication; it frequently represents a plea not to be abandoned and forgotten because of the person's terminal status. Such statements and actions may also be a form of symbolic communication, conveying emotional and spiritual pain and an attempt to make sense of inner experiences.

Secondary intervention includes a variety of forms, including individual or group therapy, electroconvulsive therapy, medication, and hospitalization. A traditional hospital practice is to place a highly suicidal individual on one-to-one, 24-hour observation and to remove all potentially harmful objects. The efficacy of this behavior is questionable, however, as it may lower the self-esteem of the depressed patient even further. It is essential to convey to the suicidal person that someone cares deeply.

Tertiary prevention, or postvention, takes place after a suicide has been completed. Its intent is to enable any survivors of the person who committed suicide to cope with the death, and to reduce the aftereffects of this traumatic event in their lives.

THE IMPACT OF SUICIDE ON SURVIVORS

In regard to suicide, according to Shneidman, the largest public health problem we face is how to relieve the effects of stress for the "survivor-victims" of suicidal death. Death by suicide is traumatic for survivors, who must deal with feelings of guilt, shame, anger, and ambiguity, along with their grief. The recent emphasis on suicides being "preventable" casts an additional burden, causing survivors to question why they were not able to prevent the act, or whether they drove the individual to suicide. Survivors also have to deal with the initial inquiry surrounding the circumstances of the death, perhaps even with being suspected of murder. Stigmatizing the survivors contributes to a feeling of shame; lack of social support heightens guilt and inhibits grief, which culminates in mourning being distorted and aborted.

Children are particularly traumatized by the suicide of a parent. They feel rejected, abandoned, and responsible. Families often respond to the stigma of suicide by creating family myths that recast events, but these do not protect the child. The family may also respond to a parental suicide by not talking about it at all, leaving the child to continually wonder what had happened.

The legacy of suicide for survivors includes reality distortion, tortured object-relations, guilt, a disturbed self-concept, impotent rage, identification with the suicide, depression, a self-destructive search for meaning, and incomplete mourning. Nevertheless, the grief process for suicide survivors appears to be similar to that of survivors of other deaths. However, because social taboos and stigmas are still attached to suicide, suicide survivors may continue to have unique problems. Often these can be addressed by specific, self-help support groups that provide the support that is often not available from family or friends.

Ideally, every community should have special bereavement counseling programs or self-help groups to aid survivors of suicide. Survivors should be helped to express feelings appropriate to the event, to grasp the reality of the suicide, and to obtain and use the help they need to work through the crisis. Professional help may or may not be necessary. Community resources that may also assist survivors include police, clergy, and funeral directors. Such postsuicide care may include three psychological stages: resuscitation—working with the family in the first 24 hours; rehabilitation—consultation with the family for the first 6 months; and renewal—a tapering off of sessions and the mourning process from 6 months on (Shneidman, Note 8).

THE HEALTH CARE PROFESSIONAL'S RESPONSE TO SUICIDE

If suicide has such a devastating effect on family and friends, how is the health care team affected? Research indicates that the staff's reaction to a patient's suicide is similar to that of family and friends. Early research on psychiatrists' responses to suicide concluded that fears concerning blame, responsibility, and inadequacy were part of their reactions. An analysis of psychiatrists' responses suggests that therapists experience guilt, heightened love, loss, and anger. The result of a recent national survey of psychologists indicated that those who had experienced a patient's suicide reported having intrusive thoughts about suicide themselves. It is important that education and training programs assist psychiatrists through such crises and provide them with support for continued personal and professional growth.

If a patient suicide occurs in the context of a treatment team, all team members may have had close relationships with the deceased and will thus feel a sense of loss. Their professional identities may be threatened, in that they "allowed" this to occur, and they may experience guilt. Staff members all experience a sense of failure, and caregivers need time to mourn and to work through feelings of anger and fear. One study showed that, after varying intensities of insecurity, the main reaction of staff members on the unit involved with a suicide was a form of overcompensation, a need to help the other patients. Another study indicated that if staff members were having difficulty discussing conflicts and disagreements before the suicide, this difficulty might be extended and escalated after the suicide.

For caregivers to be able to observe their own reactions to a patient suicide and to deal with their own depressed, anxious feelings, it is important for them to talk about these responses with each other. Informal peer contact may be the most important initial support, as the rituals of death can be supportive in terms of releasing feelings. If staff support groups are established and have been meeting regularly, staff members should be encouraged to attend these meetings to share their concerns, fears, and feelings. As intense feelings emerge, a suicide review conference held by an outside consultant might be appropriate, to reconstruct the suicide and its antecedents and to reaffirm the staff's sense of worth.

Hospital patients will also be deeply affected by a suicide within their group, and may become frightened that it could happen to them or angry at the staff for allowing it to happen. They may feel guilty about not foreseeing and preventing the suicide themselves. It is important then that a community meeting be held at which all staff and patients can discuss the event together. Such a meeting may facilitate the grieving process. The following general guidelines may help lessen the impact of a suicide death on a treatment service or facility: avoid the start and proliferation of rumors, provide for the appropriate expression of emotional responses by the patients, take special precautions with previously suicidal patients, and return to routine as quickly as appropriate, but without denying the effects of the suicide (Dunne, Note 9). As it becomes more acceptable to discuss suicide as a public health concern, it will be possible to learn more about suicide as a part of humanity.

REFERENCE NOTES

1. Gibson, P. Gay males and lesbian youth suicide. In Alcohol, Drug Abuse, and Mental Health Administration, *Report of the secretary's task force on youth suicide. Volume 3: Prevention and interventions in youth suicide*. DHHS Pub. No. (ADM) 89–1621. Washington, D.C.: U.S. Government Printing Office, 1989. Pp. 110–142.
2. Nkongho, N. O. Suicide in the elderly: A beginning investigation. *Journal of the National Black Nurses' Association*, 1988, *2*, 47–55.
3. Colt, G. W. *The enigma of suicide*. New York: Summit Books, 1991.
4. Menninger, K. *Man against himself*. New York: Harcourt Brace, 1938.
5. Stanley, M., & Stanley, B. Reconceptualizing suicide: A biological approach. *Psychiatric Annals*, 1988, *18* (11), 646–651.
6. Shneidman, E. *Deaths of man*. New York: Aronson, 1983.
7. Shneidman, E. Approaches and commonalities of suicide. In R. Diekstra, R. Maris, S. Platt, A. Schmidtke, & G. Sonneck (eds.), *Suicide and its prevention*. Leiden, The Netherlands: E. J. Brill, 1989. p. 35.
8. Shneidman, E. Approaches and commonalities of suicide, 34.
9. Dunne, E. J. A response to suicide in the mental health setting. In E. J. Dunne, J. L. McIntosh, & K. Dunn-Maxim (eds.), *Suicide and its aftermath: Understanding and counseling the survivors*. New York: Norton, 1987, pp. 186–188.

Chapter 10

Grief and Bereavement

At the end of a life, the funeral ceremony serves as the beginning of the grief and bereavement period for the survivors. The funeral reinforces the integration of the family, the community, the religious group, and the ethnic group while helping the survivors to begin their separation from the deceased through the process of mourning.

Grief and bereavement must be distinguished. Bereavement is the actual state of deprivation caused by the loss. Grief is a psychological state characterized by mental anguish. It is the response of emotional pain to the loss.

GRIEF

When people grieve, they experience conflicting behaviors and feelings: anger and apathy, for example, weight loss and weight gain, preoccupation with and suppression of memories of the deceased, the desire to discard and retain the possessions of the deceased. It is a time of great ambivalence. While the bereaved may feel lonely, often they avoid company. They both try to escape reminders of the deceased and try to keep their memory fresh. They want people to express sympathy but may resent it when it is offered.

Why do people grieve (Stroebe and Stroebe, Note 1)? Freud saw the grieving process as one that allows persons to gradually break their ties with the lost object. The person focuses on the deceased, which brings back memories, and finally begins to realize that the lost object no longer exists. Grieving is completed when the bereaved person severs the attachment to the deceased and the person can live in the present without feelings of great sadness.

According to the attachment model of grief developed by John Bowlby, grief is a form of separation anxiety. The grieving process is understood as an attempt to reestablish ties and not as a process of withdrawing from them. This theory of grief involves a search for the deceased—obviously, though, this search is extremely frustrating. Eventually the frustrated search for the deceased lessens.

This attachment theory developed from studies of children who, separated from their mother, reacted first with tears and anger but were still hopeful that their mother would return. These feelings then turned to despair, with hope and despair alternating. Finally, their memory of their mother faded.

When a loved one dies, people have the same feelings as the child separated from his or her mother. In grief, persons are continuously trying to find the lost person, going through periods of anger, yearning, and despair. Eventually the search for the deceased lessens, but people must go through these feelings if they are to recover from grief.

Another theory about the loss of a loved one is that such a loss is primarily a major source of stress. While psychoanalytic models of bereavement focus on the emotional reaction, stress models view bereavement as a stressful life event that overtaxes one's coping resources. The death of a spouse is considered one of the most stressful life events, and requires the greatest readjustment of a person's life.

The Phases of Grief

Grief consists of a number of phases, including shock and numbness; intense grief consisting of yearning, anger and guilt; and, finally, reorganization. The most immediate reaction to a death is generally a feeling of numbness. The bereaved cannot believe that the death has occurred. This stage serves as an emotional anesthetic, for to succumb to the feelings of grief at this point would be totally overwhelming. This is why the bereaved often appear to be doing so well at funerals. They may not break down; they may greet everyone with a handshake and a kind remark. In fact, however, they are acting as automatons. People admire those who react with dignity at funerals and do not break down, and the numbness of the bereaved may fool others into believing that they are doing well. After a few hours or a few days, however, the numbness should wear off, and they will enter the next phase, intense grief.

The intensity of the bereaved person's grief is not necessarily related to the degree of *love* felt for the individual who has died; rather, it is related to the degree of *feeling*, both negative and positive, for the dead person.

The writer C. S. Lewis, chronicling his grief over the death of his wife, expresses the feelings that occur in this stage: "No one ever told me that grief felt so like fear. I am not afraid, but the sensation is like being afraid. The same fluttering in the stomach, the same restlessness, the yawning. I keep on swallowing. At other times it feels like being mildly drunk, or concussed. There is a sort of invisible blanket between the world and me. I find it hard to take in what anyone says. Or perhaps, hard to want to take it in. It is so uninteresting. Yet I want the others to be about me. I dread the moments when the house is empty. If only they would talk to one another and not to me. . . . And no one ever told me about the laziness of grief. Except at my job—where the machine seems to run on much as usual—I loath the slightest effort. Not only writing but even reading a letter is too much. Even shaving. What does it matter now whether my cheek is rough or smooth? They say an unhappy man wants distractions—something to take him out of himself. Only as a dog-tired man wants an extra blanket on a cold night; he'd rather lie there shivering than get up and find one. It's easy to see why the lonely become untidy; finally, dirty and disgusting" (Lewis, Note 2).

In the first phase of intense grief, there is continued pining and searching for the deceased. The thoughts and behavior of the bereaved are focused on the lost person. Hallucinations are not uncommon. For example, in one study almost half of the bereaved people interviewed had postbereavement visual or auditory hallucinations, and several stated that they had spoken with the deceased. Although some of those interviewed questioned their own sanity, others found the hallucinations helpful.

There is also anger and guilt, which is reflected by irritability and bitterness. These feelings may be directed toward all those nearby, the doctors who took care of the deceased, God, or the deceased. The bereaved are angry at the deceased for causing such pain. Young survivors are angry because they are left alone to raise themselves or their young children. Older bereaved persons are angry about the loss of retirement plans they had made together. The bereaved may be angry at God for taking their loved one away, thinking he or she was such a good person, while so many bad people are allowed to live.

Anger may also be directed at themselves, in the form of guilt. The bereaved go through many "if only I hads." An example of this is described by author Robert Anderson, concerning the death of his wife: "I made the discovery of the very small lump in my wife's breast. I had no idea what it was. I said nothing until a solicitation from the Cancer Society listed the warning signals of cancer. For years after, I cursed my own ignorance and the negligence of all the doctors who had never taught my wife breast self-examination. For years, with hot flashes of anger and guilt, I went over and over those weeks of delay. Why didn't I mention even in passing the small lump in her breast? My brother is a doctor; why didn't I check with him? A simple phone call. For years I rewrote compulsively that scene in my head, playing it differently—I mention the lump to my wife; we go to the doctor; we are in time, and my wife is alive" (Anderson, Note 3).

During intense grief the bereaved may lapse into despair. They are disorganized, apathetic, and aimless. They have a sense of futility and emptiness, and experience a loss of patterns of interaction. These feelings of despair may come and go as the bereaved start to reorganize their lives. As they take each step in that direction, such as finding a new friend or a job, their depression gradually lifts, until the final phase, reintegration, is reached.

Reintegration, or recovery, has taken place when the bereaved are functioning normally again. A sense of the continuity of life must be reestablished. This is done, "not by ceasing to care for the dead, but by abstracting what was fundamentally important in the relationship and rehabilitating it" (Morris, Note 4). It means giving up the deceased without giving up what the deceased meant to the bereaved.

A Cleveland surgeon, Dr. George Crile, described the final stage of his grieving, a little more than a year after his wife had died: "I still live in the same house. Many of the same birds, the wood ducks and the swan, are still in our back yard. Many of the relics that Jane and I collected in our travels are about our house. But there are no ghosts. Memories that were for a time inexpressibly sad have once again become a source of deep pleasure and satisfaction. Since we know nothing of death except that it comes to all, it is not unreasonable to be sad for the person who has died. The sorrow that I once felt for myself, in my loss, now has been transformed to a rich memory of a woman I loved and the ways we traveled through the world together" (Crile, Note 5).

One never totally gets over the grief. On special occasions, such as birthdays or anniversaries, the depression may recur. The memories continue to exist, but they may become good memories.

THE SYMPTOMATOLOGY OF GRIEF AND BEREAVEMENT

Throughout the process of grieving, the bereaved may suffer from various physical symptoms. Much of what is known about the symptomatology of grief stems from the work of Erich Lindemann, a psychiatrist who treated the survivors of a nightclub fire in Boston in 1942. Many of the 200 survivors, although physically well, kept complaining of physical symptoms such as shortness of breath, insomnia, and loss of appetite. Lindemann's study of 101 bereaved persons, including survivors of the fire, found that "acute grief is a definite syndrome with psychological and somatic symptomatology (Lindemann, Note 6). Within grief, Lindemann found there was somatic distress, especially respiratory disturbance; preoccupation with the image of the deceased while feeling emotionally distant from others; guilt; hostile reactions; and loss of patterns of conduct.

Symptoms of grief fall into various categories. Affective symptoms include depression, anxiety, guilt, anger and hostility, anhedonia (loss of enjoyment or pleasure in formerly enjoyed activities), and loneliness. Behavioral manifestations of grief may take the form of self-reproach, low self-esteem, helplessness and hopelessness, a sense of unreality, suspiciousness, and interpersonal problems. Imitation of the deceased's behavior, idealization of the deceased, preoccupation with the memory of the deceased, and ambivalent feelings about the deceased are also symptoms. There may be mental impairment as well as physiological changes such as loss of appetite, sleep and energy loss, and greater susceptibility to illness.

Physical health has been shown to deteriorate during bereavement, whether measured by visits to physicians, medications taken, or reporting of one's own symptoms. For example, one study showed a significant rise in the number of visits widows made to their physicians during the first six months following the death of their spouse. Another study found that bereaved elderly persons were much more likely to be taking medication 5 to 8 months after the death than a control group of nonbereaved elderly persons.

Besides being related to ill health, is grief related to death? Do people die of broken hearts? Although grief would not be listed as a cause of death on a death certificate, epidemiological studies have shown that widows and widowers have a higher mortality rate than married people of the same sex and age. This finding cuts across cultural lines and through history. One study found an increase in the death rate of 40% during the first 6 months of bereavement. Of these deaths, 75% were attributed to heart disease, particularly coronary thromboses and arteriosclerotic heart disease. Numerous subsequent studies have confirmed that the bereaved are at a higher risk in terms of mortality.

Bereavement, then, does indeed lead to a higher death rate. Probably the best hypothesis is that the effects of grief, including feelings of hopelessness, may result in physical vulnerability. The death of a spouse, in particular, has been shown to cause the greatest amount of stress, which may cause a weakened state that results in death. The statistical relationship between grief and death does seem to suggest that people may indeed die from "broken hearts."

PATHOLOGICAL GRIEF REACTIONS

"My mother sits home alone day after day. All she does is watch television or read in between visits to Dad's grave, two, three times a week. That's what she seems to live for—those visits when she kneels down and talks to him—as if he were there, listening. Once in a while she'll go to a movie with us, or for a drive. Or let a friend come visit. But not often. I don't know. Is she losing it?" (Dersheimer, Note 7). Is the woman described having a normal reaction to the death of her spouse? Or is what she is exhibiting abnormal? Would it be considered normal at one month after the death? A year? Two years? It is very difficult to say, but studies have shown that about 15% of those who are bereaved exhibit some prolonged grief reactions.

Persons suffering from abnormal grief reactions exaggerate the normal aspects of grief; they seem unable to resolve the conflicts of grief as most other persons do. The depression, panic, guilt, and ill health that are felt in these distorted forms of grief do not differ in kind, but rather in duration and intensity, from normal grief reactions.

Patterns of abnormal grief reactions may include the following:

Delayed grief. The bereaved feels little sorrow and continues on with life, acting very busy and being very calm. This may last a few weeks or even longer. Suddenly, the grief may be triggered by the loss of some object, such as a wristwatch; or it may be triggered when the circumstances surrounding the death are recalled. A person with a very severe reaction to a recent death may also be grieving for another person who died years before.

Inhibited grief. The bereaved never feels grief. Perhaps only if other symptoms develop, including such physical conditions as ulcerative colitis, asthma, or rheumatoid arthritis, should this be viewed as a pathological form of grieving, for it does appear that not all people necessarily or inevitably feel distress when they are bereaved.

Chronic grief. The grieving continues; the bereaved person can never get beyond the intense yearning for the one who has died, the anger, guilt, and despair. One man was reported as still actively grieving for his wife after three years, reminiscing constantly over their marriage, idealizing their relationship, and still unable to look after himself.

Bereavement may be prolonged when society does not recognize a person's right to grieve, as in the case of gay men who have experienced the death of their lover from AIDS. This has been called disenfranchised grief.

Which bereaved persons are most likely to have a poor outcome? Although theorists have listed more than ten variables that affect the outcome of bereavement (including age, sex, social class, prior grief experiences, religiosity, personality of the bereaved, type of relationship, timeliness, mode of death, cause of death, and quality of social supports), there is clear evidence only for the following factors:

- Men have more difficulty adjusting than women.

- Younger bereaved persons are at greater risk than older bereaved persons.
- Overdependent and ambivalent relationships generally lead to poor grief outcomes.
- Social support and perceived social support are important in defining those bereaved persons who are at high risk.

ANTICIPATORY GRIEF

When people expect the death of someone close, they may begin to experience their grief in advance. There is disagreement in the research data about whether this anticipatory grief is helpful or not. Why are the findings contradictory? The answer, in part, is that the studies define anticipatory grief differently, examine different age groups, and measure outcome at a different time.

Obviously the sudden death of an elderly person under natural circumstances would elicit different reactions than the sudden and violent death of a younger person. Furthermore, a forewarning of loss is not the same as anticipating grief. The survivor of a person who was ill prior to dying may have grieved in anticipation, or the bereaved may have denied the oncoming death. One study on anticipatory grief showed that those who had the best outcome were the survivors of those who had had an illness lasting less than six months, as compared with survivors of someone who had either died suddenly or been ill for a longer period of time.

It appears that anticipatory grief is not inherently positive or negative, especially in regard to the ambivalence that is felt when a loved one is dying. While a period of anticipatory grief allows the mourner to feel some grief in advance of the loss, it also may permit the negative side of the ambivalence of grief to be experienced over a long period of time. If the patient is not being told that he or she is dying, and some closed or mutual pretense awareness exists, it becomes difficult to work out these ambivalent feelings. Furthermore, throughout anticipatory grief the survivor must maintain hope; if he or she does not, the survivor may be viewed as not having loved the dying person. Anticipatory grief may lead survivors to feel that they gave up hope too soon.

Anticipating the Death of a Child

Anticipatory parental mourning is a process in which emotional attachment to the dying child is gradually relinquished. Such mourning is really a set of processes consisting of a growing realization by the parents that their child's death is inevitable, with an alternation of hope and despair as this realization deepens. Then the feelings of grief, which began as intense undifferentiated responses, eventually become less acute, and the parents develop some perspective about their child's impending death, acknowledging that the child's life has been worthwhile and that life will continue for them after the child has died. This is followed by some degree of detachment. While the parents still offer love and security to their dying child, they begin to reinvest in relationships that will continue after the child dies. Finally, there is memorialization, the development of a positive mental image of the child that will endure after her or his death and remembering the child in generalities rather than in terms of specific behaviors.

Although anticipatory grief may be helpful for parents, it may also result in family members separating from the child before he or she has died. This can occur when the dying process extends over a long time, or if the child has an unexpected late remission. Parents may be upset to find that they have withdrawn from their child before the actual death. Both they and the child may need support from health care staff so that the child does not become isolated.

Caregivers' Role

During the period of anticipatory grief, patients and all those involved in their care, including the health care team, need as much support as possible. The patient and the family are attempting to cope with uncertainties that lead to feelings of ambivalence, anger, and guilt, and conflict among family members. When the patient is a child, a lack of understanding between the parents can adversely affect their entire future. Premature mourning and the withdrawal of the family isolates the patient and frustrates the health care team if they do not understand the underlying dynamics. At the same time, the professional caregivers are also struggling with their sense of impotence and with having to shift from curing to caring. Their anger can easily be projected onto the family for "not caring," when they are actually unable to deal with their own feelings about "not curing."

The use of support groups to help families discuss what must be faced and how to accomplish this is an extremely effective method of promoting better understanding during a period of anticipatory grief. It is particularly beneficial if members of the health care team can participate in the process, or at least are informed of it. It is desirable to encourage family involvement during the period of anticipatory grief. While each family member may be threatened by a sense of loss, each can be helped to enhance an awareness and understanding of eath other's relationship. Some adaptational tasks are to remain involved with the patient as well as to separate from him or her, to adapt to role changes, to bear the effects of grief, to come to some terms with the reality of impending loss, and to say good-bye. Obviously the first two tasks, which sound mutually exclusive, require understanding and creative therapeutic intervention. These techniques, however, need not be complex. For example, a family member can be encouraged to include the patient in all family decisions and communications. Often family members will tell the health care staff what they feel a patient needs and must gently be reminded to ask the patient's preference. Similarly, families can be given "permission" by staff not to visit. At the Victoria General Hospice progam (Victoria, Canada), one day is set aside as "relatives' day off" (Lebow, Note 8).

PARENTS' GRIEF

The death of a child, no matter what age, is one of the most traumatic experiences a family will ever have to endure. During the initial phase of numbness and shock, the parents may view their child's death as an unreal experience that may be denied. Parents may also be flooded with feelings of anger, guilt, rage, and frustration. The most important response of caregivers at this point is one of caring, being available to listen to the parents. Parents may also need practical help in making such decisions as whom to call to notify of the death and how to arrange for a funeral home.

The parents' numbness and shock may persist as a protective shield for days or weeks, but gradually it will give way to the period of intense grief. This time is painful and depressing. Grieving family members may find that they were isolated from the community while their child was dying and that they isolated for a time after the child's death. Friends and relatives may avoid the family, perhaps even more so if the child has died from a disease such as AIDS, which society fears. Parents often want to talk about the child's death, however, and they want company. Single parents may feel particularly alone. One single parent wrote, "I had no one to share the experience with; no one to even enter my house of silence" (Wyler, Note 9).

In one study of families mourning the death of a child, it was found that while several of the mothers expressed an intense need to talk about the child and the death, their husbands were unable to speak of it and even refused to allow the child's name to be mentioned. Parents need to understand that their partners, while experiencing feelings of grief and loss, may express their feelings in unique ways. Fathers are often put in the role of the strong and silent one, even if they have painful and sad feelings and would like to express them. One parent may have a need to cope with grief through sexual intimacy, whereas the other parent may find this aspect of the relationship of little interest at this time.

Parents also may not be in the same phase of grieving at the same time. A mother, ofen because of her usually closer and more continuous contact with the dying child, may have worked through anticipatory grieving feelings and be in more of a stage of detachment than the father, who may still be experiencing tremendous feelings of anger and guilt. Generally, difficulties between parents arise when one parent expects the other to respond to grief in the same way and at the same time. Parents may need help in understanding that each of them may grieve differently over the death of their child.

During the period of intense grieving, parents may experience physical distress, including poor appetite, insomnia, irritability, muscular aches and pain, and digestive problems. Caregivers can help bereaved parents try to maintain appropriate eating, sleeping, and exercise patterns. Some parents may turn to the use of drugs and alcohol to avoid the pain of grief. There is a real danger of such use changing into abuse, which can lead to addiction. If substance abuse occurs, caregivers need to refer the parent to an appropriate treatment center for help.

Reorganization in the grieving process becomes more evident as parents begin to feel that life does indeed still contain some pleasures, some degree of comfort. They are able to enjoy again aspects of living that they enjoyed prior to their child's death, such as sports, watching TV, reading a good book, taking a vacation. Parents may feel guilty about "having fun," however, and may need to be reassured that it is quite acceptable to begin to enjoy life again.

Caregivers must remember that reorganization is not recovery. Parents say that they never recover from the loss of a child. For many people, the pain of grief can still be evoked years after a child's death—the pain may be less sharp and not last as long, but it can still be there.

ROLE CHANGES AFTER THE DEATH OF A SPOUSE

After the death of a spouse, there are major changes in the life of the survivor. Once bereaved wives and husbands begin recovering from their grief, they are faced with being widows and widowers. But they don't know the rules for these roles. Widowhood is generally viewed as a temporary state, but a temporary state on the way to what? When does one stop being a widow and become a single person?

Widows and widowers face specific problems in no longer being married and in being alone in a couples-oriented society. In one study of widows, over 50% agreed with the statement: "One problem of being a widow is feeling like a fifth wheel." Younger widows may now find themselves perceived as a sexual threat by many of their friends; they may feel that the other women are jealous of them when their husbands are around. One attractive widow in her 40s, for example, reported how her relationship with her sister-in-law changed after her husband's death. Before, she had always greeted her brother-in-law and his wife with a hug and kiss. Now when she went to kiss her brother-in-law, the sister-in-law gives her a dirty look.

Dating and sex become issues for the bereaved. Widows, especially, are not supposed to have any interest in sex. For example, one young widow reported: "My husband and I had a good sex life. Since he passed away, I've lived like a virgin. My minister was evasive when I mentioned my sense of frustration. He gave me that 'Now, now my dear' response, but I got his message: 'Respectable women shouldn't have such desires, it isn't nice.'"

When does it become all right for a widow to begin dating again? When is it all right to have sex again? Although some would argue that the answers are best left to the individual, having some societal guidelines would help alleviate the guilt a widow or widower may feel when beginning to date. As one widow asked, "When it is all right for me to take off my wedding band?"

Widows and widowers of different ages face different specific problems. From age 30 to 54, the death of a spouse usually means that the income of the family drops substantially. There may be children who must be taken care of, yet there is a lack of inexpensive daycare. The widow age 55 to 65 is not likely to have dependent children, but she is not yet eligible for Social Security benefits, which may mean that she will become poor. It is also harder for her to reenter the job market if she has not worked outside the home in a number of years. Although she may want to date, and eventually remarry, there is a paucity of eligible men. Finally at age 65 and older, the widow may be left relatively isolated.

The younger widower must now become more aware of his children's social and emotional needs, and often realizes how dependent he was on his spouse for maintaining the emotional balance in the family. The older widower may not be prepared to take care of himself, because his wife was always responsible for the housework and cooking. If he is retired, he no longer has either of the two primary roles in our society: worker and spouse. As a result, he may begin to feel worthless. The one major advantage a widower has over a widow is that it is easier for him to remarry: there is a 5 to 1 ratio of widows to widowers.

CAREGIVERS' ROLES WITH THE BEREAVED

Although studies indicate that persons who are bereaved represent a higher-risk population with regard to physical and emotional illness and even death, relatively few programs are available to provide support through this difficult period. Everyone assumes that the grieving individual will "get over it." Certainly the vast majority do. But the health care team and the community can facilitate grieving and provide support to enhance the bereaved persons' continued growth and development. The bereaved person often needs someone who will be able to sit and listen. This sounds simplistic, but we as caregivers often feel the need to give advice and counsel, sometimes to escape our own feelings of helplessness. This "rush to help" can prevent us from hearing what the bereaved individual says is needed. Our cultural emphasis on competency, strength, and adequacy can prevent the bereaved from experiencing the emotions necessary for appropriate resolution of grief.

Repetition is necessary for the mastery of loss. The bereaved require repeated opportunities to verbalize their feelings as they attempt to make sense of their loss; they need to ask the unanswerable "why?" before acceptance of the loss is reached. One father, in discussing his responses to his daughter's death, explained: "I needed the opportunity to talk, over and over and over, to repeat and repeat and repeat and repeat. And to have somebody be able to listen to that" (Hallinger, Note 10). This process begins as soon as the individual is told that death has occurred.

Currently the majority of deaths in this country occur in institutional settings. The health care team, pressured by the demands of the setting and members' own sense of failure, often allocates little time with family members after a patient has died. Even when death is still expected, families respond with shock, numbness, and dismay. Physicians, nurses, and social workers often feel impatient with this response, and a common reaction is to withdraw. Some members of the health care team should remain available to assist family members as they incorporate their initial shock. Often this is perceived as a social work task, since the social worker is not responsible for ongoing, direct patient care. If possible, provision should also be made for some room where privacy is ensured. Also, whether or not they were present at the exact moment of death, family members usually require reassurance that "everything was done."

Each family member has an individual response to death, and the caregiver must carefully observe and respond to these needs. A few common themes emerge during this period. First, there is ambivalence about seeing the person immediately following death. Second, there is confusion about how one tells other family members and begins preparation for funeral arrangements. Family members may well look to the caregiver as the "expert."

If members of the health care team have had an extended, intensive relationship with the deceased and the family, attending the funeral or memorial service has salutary effects for everyone. The family welcomes the recognition of their needs and the respect for their dead, and the caregiver has an opportunity to "say good-bye."

Grief Counseling

To help facilitate the grieving process, the bereaved may get involved in grief counseling. William Worden presents a framework for such counseling (Worden, Note 11). Four tasks that the bereaved must complete correspond to the four goals for grief counseling. The grieving person must accept the reality of the loss, experience the pain of grief, adjust to an environment in which the deceased is missing, and withdraw emotional energy and reinvest it in another relationship. The corresponding goals in grief counseling are to increase the reality of the loss, to help the counselee deal with both expressed and latent feelings, to help the counselee overcome various impediments to readjustment after the loss, and to encourage the counselee to make a healthy emotional withdrawal from the deceased and to feel comfortable reinvesting that emotion in another relationship.

To accomplish these goals, there are a number of guidelines for the counselor: (1) to help the survivor actualize the loss by allowing the survivor to talk about it; (2) to help the survivor identify and express feelings, such as anger, guilt, anxiety, helplessness, and sadness; (3) to assist in living without the deceased by helping the survivor make decisions; (4) to facilitate emotional withdrawal from the deceased by encouraging the bereaved to form new relationships; (5) to provide time to grieve by recognizing that grieving takes time and that certain dates, such as birthdays and holidays, may be difficult; (6) to interpret normal behavior by reassuring the bereaved that what they are going through is not "craziness"; (7) to allow for individual differences; (8) to provide continuing support; (9) to examine defenses and coping styles, particularly those which may be hurtful, such as using alcohol; and (10) to identify pathology in the grief response and refer people to intensive therapy as appropriate.

In addition to grief counseling, the bereaved may choose to become part of a self-help group. Such programs are run by volunteers who are willing to use their own experiences to help others learn to deal with their transition, to prevent problems at a later time, and to look forward to the future.

REFERENCE NOTES

1. For a discussion of theories of grieving see Stroebe, W., & Stroebe, M. *Bereavement and health*. Cambridge, England: Cambridge University Press, 1989.
2. Lewis, C. S. *A grief observed*. New York: Seabury Press, 1961, pp. 1–2.
3. Anderson, R. Notes of a survivor. In S. Troup & W. Green (eds.), *The patient, death and the family*. New York: Scribners, 1944, p. 10.
4. Morris, P. *Loss and change*. New York: Pantheon Books, 1974, p. 34.
5. Crile, G. Memorial service. In A. Kutscher (ed.), *Death and bereavement*. Springfield, Ill.: Charles C. Thomas, 1969, p. xxiii.
6. Lindemann, E. Symptomatology and management of acute grief. *American Journal of Psychiatry*, 1944, *101*, 141.
7. Dersheimer, R. *Counseling the bereaved*. New York: Pergamon Press, 1990, p. 31.
8. Lebow, G. Facilitating adaptation in anticipatory mourning. *Social Casework*, 1976, *57* (7), 458–465.
9. Wyler, J. Grieving alone: A single mother's loss." *Issues in Comprehensive Pediatric Nursing*, 1988, *12* (4), 301.
10. Hallinger, R. Parents of murdered children need special grief work. *Thanatology Today*, 1988, *2*, 2.
11. Worden, W. *Grief counseling and grief therapy*. New York: Springer Publishers, 1982.

Death from a Cross-Cultural Perspective

Serena Nanda

> *Today is a good day to die, for all the things of my life*
> *are present.*
>
> —*Crazy Horse, leader of the Oglala Sioux*

Every culture provides a way for its members to think about and respond to death. Death is set off by rituals that are based on culturally patterned beliefs and social institutions, and culture plays an important role in shaping not only the beliefs and practices regarding death and dying, but also the motions elicited by these events. We can use our knowledge of death beliefs and practices as a way of understanding a society. In the United States, for example, death is probably the most intensely experienced of all human crises, yet it is also the one least talked about. This, in itself, is an indication of our anxiety about it.

The universality of beliefs and rituals centering on death and the fate of the human soul demonstrate our human preoccupation with dying and the decaying human body. All human societies attempt to control death by symbolically imposing order on the universe and thus giving purpose to life. Almost every human culture incorporates the belief that death is not the end of the person, but is rather a passage from the world of the living to another world, or spirit realm. This belief offers an active role for those who have died, viewing them as either potential enemies that require careful handling or potential guardians who help the living. In American society today, our biomedical perspective shapes our view that death occurs because humans are genetically programmed to die. Yet Americans, like others, are uncomfortable with the idea that death means the end of all individual awareness.

BELIEFS ABOUT THE AFTERLIFE

Most cultures are explicit about beliefs that death is only a transition from one social status to another, and that the dead remain in touch with the living. Among the Gikuyu of East Africa, for instance, the dead are an important element in everyday life. Because the Gikuyu believe that the spirits of the dead can be pleased or displeased by the behavior of the living, and can act in a beneficent or spiteful manner, the ceremony of communing with the ancestral spirits is constantly observed in Gikuyu society.

In societies in which concepts of time are different from our own, and where past, present, and future are merged, beliefs about the continuous relationship of the dead with the living pose no intellectual problem. A dramatic example of this kind of belief is the "Dreamtime" belief of the indigenous peoples of Australia. The Dreamtime is the long-ago time when the ancestors created all the animate and inanimate things in the cosmos, including the aboriginal people themselves. In all the important Australian ceremonies, the Dreamtime is recreated through the telling of legends and ritual performances. The aboriginal Australians believe that each person's spirit came from a clan pool of spirits, entering his or her mother's womb at the time of conception and returning to the common pool after death. To repay this debt of creation to the ancestors, the Australians commemorate the events of the Dreamtime in their great initiation ceremonies, when, they believe, they become ancestors.

A similar belief connecting the living and the dead exists among the Central Inuit people of the Arctic. There, the name of the last person to die in a settlement is given to the first child born thereafter, and the child is considered to be the reincarnation of the dead person.

Cultural beliefs also differ in picturing what the afterworld looks like. In some cases, it is described as an earthly paradise, providing humans with all that they lack in this world. In other cases, the afterworld closely resembles life on earth. Among the Tikopia of Polynesia, for example, the soul makes courtesy visits to ancestral spirits, guided by the same rules of etiquette that hold on earth. And, unlike the Christian belief that all souls will be equal in Heaven, in Tikopian belief the souls of the dead keep their earthly status. The system of clan dwellings after death, the special position of chiefs and ritual leaders, and the role of the married and the unmarried all broadly reflect living Tikopian society. This reproduction of the social system reinforces the belief that not only the individual but also, more important, the society will continue after its present members have died.

The social and psychological functions of these widespread beliefs are not difficult to understand. Societies regard themselves as ongoing systems, and the death of any member threatens the very existence of society. Society refuses to consider death an irrevocable end to life; it considers it to be also the beginning of a new existence. Thus, the idea of death is linked with that of resurrection—separation followed by a new integration.

Beliefs in an afterlife can be seen as an answer to the threat that death makes against the social system. In Western thought, life is identified with individuality, and death is threatening because it ends this differentiation. Hence the importance of grave monuments, which identify the dead as individuals. Science is influenced by and makes use of this cultural anxiety, as archeologists use grave goods and skeletal data to reconstruct as many of the individual features of the dead as possible. Contemporary

Western beliefs, which emphasize the break between past and present, the separation of the living and the dead, and the individual and the soul at the expense of the continuation of the community and the universe, stand nearly by themselves. Other societies emphasize continuity—between past and present, living and dead, individual and community.

ATTITUDES TOWARD PAIN, DYING, AND DEATH

Very little has been written about response to pain in other cultures and the attitudes of actual individuals to death and dying, or about the milieu of the dying person and how this affects their attitudes toward death. It does seem, however, that there is a cultural dimension to such emotional and behavioral responses.

A cultural dimension to pain experiences has been noticed in the case of Alaskan Indians, for example, who are reported to tolerate extreme pain very calmly for brief periods, provided that it is accompanied by the hope of fast relief and recovery, but tolerate pain very poorly if the prognosis is unknown. A study of Samoan patients with severe burns, hospitalized in the United States, found that they were extraordinarily stoic in the face of their great pain, and that the emotional trauma usually observed in severe burn cases was absent both among the patients and their families.

Among Hindu Indians, the attitude toward pain is related to the attitude toward death, which is itself influenced by such religious beliefs as karma, or fate. Hindus believe that just as the quality of one's life is shaped by one's deeds in a previous life, so too is the quality of one's death shaped by how well one has behaved in this life. Those people who believe that they have acted rightly in their present life can accept the fact of death. Unlike in the United States, where every effort is made to prolong life—even when it involves permanent, debilitating, and agonizing pain with little hope of cure—in India, older persons are taught to prepare positively for death, and to prefer an early death to a long life of pain and suffering. Death is openly talked about among family members, and the acceptance of death's inevitability permits older people to prepare for it emotionally and spiritually.

According to Islamic belief, the dying person should ideally be surrounded by friends and relatives. Islam imposes responsibilities on a person who knows death is imminent: he or she must ask forgiveness of God and other people, and forgive others as well. Debts must be paid off or arrangements made to have them paid by others, or creditors must be asked for forgiveness. A dying person must also make a will. The dying must take care of their body in certain ways, cleaning their teeth and body and putting on clean clothes. The dying person must recite the Quran. It is the responsibility of those near the dying individual to remind him or her of these and other duties.

What seems apparent from these examples of dying in other cultures is that, regardless of the specific treatment of the dying person, he or she dies within the mileu of the community. At the moment of death, if not during the long illness that may precede it, the community responds to what is a matter of public, not merely private, concern. Dying people in other cultures die in the midst of life that is going on around them.

GRIEF REACTIONS: COMMON EXPERIENCES

Because people everywhere build long-term, interdependent relationships that produce feelings of attachment and caring, the end of these relationships produces emotional distress and disorganization in every culture. In spite of cultural differences, then, there are some universal, or at least very widespread, individual and social reactions to death. In all cultures, as in the United States, people react to death with expression of emotions— sadness, emptiness, fear, and anger.

Of all the expressions of grief associated with death, crying, or "wailing," is the most common. The intensity of emotion expressed in some non-Western societies may seem shocking to Americans, where outward "bearing up" and emotional self-restraint are important values in funeral behavior. In the following scene among the Warramunga of Australia, a group of participants and spectators was leaving the area where a totemic ceremony has just been celebrated, when a piercing cry suddenly came from the camp where a man was dying:

At once the whole company commenced to run as fast as they could while most of them commenced to howl. . . . Some of the men . . . sat down bending their heads forward . . . while they wept and moaned. . . . Some of the women . . . were lying prostrate on the body, while others were standing or kneeling around, digging the sharp ends of their yarn sticks into the crown of their heads, from which the blood streamed down over their faces, while all the time keeping up a loud, continuous wail. Many of the men, rushing up to the spot, threw themselves upon the body. . . . To one side three men began wailing loudly . . . and in a minute or two another man of the same (totemic group) rushed on to the group yelling and brandishing a stone knife. Reaching the camp, he suddenly gashed both thighs deeply, cutting right across the muscles, and unable to stand, fell down into the middle of the group. The (dying) man did not actually die until late in the evening. As soon as he had given up his last breath, the same scene was re-enacted, only this time the wailing was still louder, and men and women, seized by a veritable frenzy, were rushing about cutting themselves with knives and sharp-pointed sticks, the women battering one another's heads with fighting clubs (Huntington and Metcalf, Note 1).

Every culture has norms about the kinds and intensity of emotions that are appropriate at death. While some religious traditions, such as Islam, censure loud wailing at death because it contests the idea of God's omnipotence and wisdom, many cultures other than our own permit or even encourage intense emotional expressions of grief, which have a positive cathartic effect on the survivors closely related to the deceased. Structured, collective, yet powerful emotional expression is noticeable by its absence in grief behavior in the United States. Because it appears that working through grief and the resumption of a normal life take less time when intense emotional expression is collectively displayed as part of funeral ceremonies, we should not be surprised to find that Americans experience grief longer and take longer to resume a normal pattern of life than people in some other cultures do.

Social Status of the Deceased

In considering the expression of grief in other cultures, we may have to look at the social position of the dead or dying person. Although most Americans would not want to admit that the mourning of a person's death should or does correspond to the individual's sex, age, or socioeconomic status, this does appear to be the case in all societies. In societies with high infant mortality, for example, a child's death does not occasion the extended ceremonies that take place for adults.

The absence of public and ritualized grieving for children should not be taken to mean that their deaths do not cause intense emotions. A study of the impact of children's death on mothers among the Shona of Zimbabwe indicated that although few of the 124 women interviewed had public funerals for their very young children who had died, all but one reported experiencing grief over the death. Furthermore, several of the mothers specifically mentioned the contradiction between the cultural taboo against public crying for a stillborn child or an infant under 6 months, and their own personal intense grief experience.

In addition to age, social status and the relationship to the deceased account for variations in the expression of grief or mourning behavior. In Chinese culture, this aspect is formalized in the *wu fu*, or five degrees of mourning, which depend on whether the deceased was a spouse (with a wife mourning her husband longer than the reverse), a grandparent, a sibling, an aunt or uncle, or a more distant relative. For the death of a very elderly person, joy rather than grief is expressed to celebrate the person's having lived to a ripe old age.

Appropriate Feelings

In our society, feelings of loss and sadness are considered the most appropriate ones to express at death, and feelings of anger are considered out of place. In other societies, however, feelings of anger and aggression are frequently expressed in grief.

It is not difficult for professionals to understand why anger and aggression might accompany bereavement, perhaps even predominating over sorrow, when a very near and loved person has died. From a social point of view, the question is how to prevent the anger and aggression of the bereaved from damaging the social relations of the survivors. Most societies try to channel the anger and aggression of grief along nondestructive paths. Here, ritual activities and specialists play an important role by providing predictable and correct activities for the bereaved to engage in, minimizing the frustration that might come from not knowing what to do when death occurs. Ritual activities also keep the close survivors busy—often praying, singing, dancing, even engaging in sexual orgies that may direct aggressive energies into channels that do not result in harmful attacks on other persons. Ritual specialists are also useful in defining the often ambiguous feelings of bereaved persons as sorrow rather than anger; ritual itself may channel anger and aggression toward institutionalized targets—for example, out-groups—or oneself.

In complex, socially stratified societies, where religious obligations in burial and mourning entail expense, anger toward one's poverty and toward established religious institutions may be a prominent emotion elicited by the death of a family member. In *A Death in the Sanchez Family*, author Oscar Lewis exposes the wide range of emotions that come into play as a poor Mexican family tries to organize a decent burial for one of its members. As Lewis says in his introduction, "For the poor, death is almost as great a hardship as life itself."

Another cultural context in which aggression is elaborated as a response to death is in those groups where no deaths, or few deaths, are considered "natural." Among the Dobu, who live on an island in the Western Pacific, there is perpetual distrust of everyone in the community except for a very small group of people. The first questions raised by the kin of the sick person is, "Who is to blame?" Every Dobu death is believed to have been caused by witchcraft, sorcery, poisoning, suicide, or assault. Every person on the island knows the spells to cause specific diseases or death. Therefore, when someone dies, the kin use various divination techniques to discover whose grudge killed their relative. Often the most suspicion falls on those who were the closest to the deceased before he or she died. Although most societies are not as suspicious as the Dobu, the projection of blame onto others for death seems to be quite widespread. Perhaps this projection serves the purpose of directing the anger and aggression of the deceased person's kin into culturally acceptable channels.

Suicide

"In some [Eskimo] tribes, an old man wants his oldest son or favorite daughter to be the one to put the string around his neck and hoist him to his death. This was always done at the height of a party where good things were being eaten, where everyone—including the one who was about to die—felt happy and gay, and which would end with . . . dancing to chase out the evil spirits. At the end of his performance, he would give a special rope . . . to the 'executioner,' who then placed it over the beam of the roof of the house and fastened it around the neck of the old man. Then the two rubbed noses, and the young man pulled the rope. Everybody in the house either helped or sat on the end of the rope so as to have the honor of bringing the old suffering one to the Happy Hunting Grounds where there would always be light and plenty of game of all kinds" (Freuchen, Note 2).

As this description of an Inuit (Eskimo) suicide suggests, the attitudes, frequency, and methods of self-inflicted death are all influenced by culture. Suicide is a socially meaningful action, but its meanings are different in different societies. Certainly, the almost universally negative reaction to suicide in the United States, which is related to our prolonging of life at any price as well as our fear of death, is not a reaction found in all cultures.

The Inuit suicide contrasts with suicide in our own society, where every type of control is brought to bear on keeping the attempted suicide alive. Cultural meanings are evoked ("Suicide is a sin"); familial pressures are applied ("How could you abandon your spouse and children?"); psychological and even legal forces—attempted suicide is a crime—are mobilized to prevent the individual from attempting suicide. An interesting point is that although active control and initiative are encouraged in almost every aspect of American life and culture, in death the individual is expected to remain passive.

It appears that there are similar motives for suicide in very different cultures. In African cultures, for example, suicide appears to be motivated by such factors as domestic strife and the loss, or fear of loss, of social status, much as it is in the United States. In addition, African societies also have motives for suicide largely unknown here, such as the fear of ghosts or other supernatural figures who are believed to have the power to cause one's death.

The impact of the supernatural in matters of suicide also relates to voodoo death, or death by sorcery or witchcraft. Because some witchcraft victims simply resign themselves to dying once they know that they have had a spell cast on them, Western observers might interpret this as subintentioned death, that is, a form of death in which the deceased plays an indirect, covert, partial, or unconscious role in his or her own demise.

The most vivid descriptions of this type of death come from Australian aboriginal societies in which the sorcerer is believed to work his magic by pointing a bone at the victim: "The man who discovers that he is being boned . . . stands aghast, with his eyes staring at the treacherous pointer, and with his hands lifted as though to ward off the lethal medium, which he imagines is pouring into his body. His cheeks blanch and his eyes become glassy and the expression of his face becomes horribly distorted. . . . His body begins to tremble and the muscles twist involuntarily. He sways backwards and falls to the ground, and after a short time appears to be in a swoon; but soon after he writhes as if in mortal agony, and, covering his face with his hands, begins to moan. After a while he becomes very composed and crawls to his worley. From this time onwards he sickens and frets, refusing to eat and keeping aloof from the daily affairs of the tribe. Unless help is forthcoming in the shape of a countercharm . . . his death is only a matter of a comparatively short time" (Cannon, Note 3).

THE RITUALS OF DEATH: FUNERALS AND MOURNING

In all cultures death raises a series of problems pertaining to the obligations imposed on the survivors: the corpse must be looked after; the deceased must be placed in a new status; the roles vacated by the deceased must be filled and their property disposed of; the solidarity of the group must be reaffirmed; and the bereaved must be comforted and reestablished in their relationships to others.

Mortuary or funeral rites have many functions: they give meaning and sanction to the separation of the dead person from the living; they help effect the transition of the soul to another, otherworldly realm; they assist in the incorporation of the spirit to its new existence. In most societies, the kin and the entire community are prominent in these rituals. Through performing mortuary rituals, as well as through observing mourning behavior, community members have a vital role in realizing a communal goal—the removal of the dead person's spirit so that it will not menace the living. This is most frequently accomplished by the practice of secondary treatment of the corpse.

Secondary treatment is the regular and socially sanctioned removal of some or all of the relics of the person from the place of temporary storage to a permanent resting place. It is one of the most frequent elements in death rituals in other cultures. Among the Berawan of Borneo, for example, there are two major ceremonies, separated by a period of anywhere from eight months to five years. The first ceremony begins immediately after death. The corpse is displayed for a day or two, until it has been viewed by all the close kin. It is then put into a coffin or a large jar. At the end of a week, this is removed for temporary storage and is placed either in the longhouse or on a platform in the graveyard. At the second ceremony, people come from all over. The coffin or jar is brought to a small shed on the longhouse veranda. Every evening for about a week there is a party near where the jar of bones is kept. The bones are then transferred to their final resting place, either in a wooden mausoleum or in the niche of a massive, carved wooden post.

In societies like that of the Berawan, where secondary treatment is practiced, death is not seen as immediate. Rather, there is a period during which the individual is believed to be neither alive nor finally dead. During this period, the process of decomposition of the corpse may be said to represent the liminality, or transition period, of the soul. As the body decays and is in an impermanent and miserable state of rotting, so the soul too, is in its impermanent and restless position, wandering around the living, perhaps seeking to pull others after it. It is at this time the corpse is most feared, and the fear of the corpse mirrors the fear of the spirit of the dead person. After the secondary treatment (burial or cremation of the bones), the soul of the deceased is considered to have reached and been integrated into the afterworld and is no longer feared. Secondary treatment rituals often are the official end to the mourning period and mark the point at which a surviving spouse may remarry.

Another contrast between death rituals in our own society and in many others is the important role played by symbolic demonstrations of the themes of sexuality, fertility, and the continuation of life at funerals. These values are noticeable by their absence in America, where funerals are generally subdued, if not gloomy, affairs. In Madagascar, by contrast, among the Bara people, funerals involve "bawdy and drunken revelry enjoined upon the guests." An important part of the funeral procession, during which the coffin is carried from the house to a cave in the hills, is a chase in which young girls run after the youths carrying the coffin, followed by adults and, finally, the family cattle. Only boys who have had sexual experience can participate in this, and it is viewed as essentially a sexual contest between boys and girls for possession of the corpse. About halfway up the mountain, the procession halts, the cattle are stampeded around the coffin, and the young men compete with each other in cattle wrestling. Then the procession begins again. Disorderly conduct of various kinds is essential at Bara funerals and secondary burial ceremonies. Toward this end, rum is served, and dancing, contests involving cattle, and sexual activities are part of the festivities. Such festivities have important psychological and social functions related to resuming normal behavior.

While death rituals vary, as we have seen, according to the social status of the deceased, there is also an important underlying similarity or unity in death rituals across wide cultural and historical lines. Traditionally, in China, for example, where the correct performance of death rituals was of concern to both commoners and elites, funeral practices throughout society consisted of many common elements: public notification of death, donning of mourning clothes by the kin of the deceased, ritualized bathing of the corpse, the provision of food, goods, and money to the deceased, preparation of a soul tablet for the domestic altar, music to accompany the corpse and settle the spirit, the sealing of the corpse into an airtight coffin, and the expulsion of the corpse from the community. The Chinese state took the initiative in setting proper norms for the death ritual, and with the advent of printing, distributed pamphlets on the correct ritual far and wide across the empire.

Mourning rituals function to integrate persons, particularly the spouse of the deceased, into society. Undoubtedly, one of the important functions of a mourning period is to limit the grief of the bereaved so that they may eventually return to more or less normal patterns of behavior. Just as funerary rites provide a passage in status for the deceased, so mourning rites provide a passage in status for the survivors. In all societies bereavement is not expected to be permanent. To the extent that a culturally defined mourning ritual exists, it both supports the expression of grief in a culturally approved way and limits the period of grief by limiting the period of mourning.

Two widespread mourning practices are marking and isolating the close survivors of the deceased. Isolation involves a limited time period during which close and specified kin of the deceased are kept apart from the rest of society. Isolation occurs more frequently for widows than for widowers, and more for spouses than for parents of a dead child or for adult children of aged parents. This suggests that grief may be less when the deceased is economically marginal. Where concepts of pollution or certain taboos must be observed involving isolation or marking, it is most frequently the spouse who is most subject to them. Among the Tlingit, for example, all those who participated in touching the corpse in preparation for its cremation were under taboos of various sorts; but the deceased's widow, in particular, "was the prisoner of taboo." She was not allowed to speak for 12 days after the death of her husband, nor allowed to do work of any kind. She was not allowed to use a knife or cup. Her clothing and bedding were taken from her and burned along with the clippings of her hair, which she had cut for the cremation. A rock was placed on her bed, which was supposed to assure her next husband of a long life. A rope was placed around her waist, and this was said to guarantee long life for her relatives. These customs clearly imply a responsibility in the widow for the life and well-being of her closest kin, as well as the expectation that she would remarry.

In a cross-cultural survey of mourning behavior, it was found that the mourning of spouses for each other involves the most ritual and emotional expression in most societies. It is also true cross-culturally that women are permitted, and perhaps expected, to behave more emotionally than men when a death occurs. There are several possible explanations for this. Men may actually experience a loss less deeply, since women in their roles as wives and mothers may experience stronger attachments than men do in their roles. Another explanation may be that women are more strongly coerced than men by the normative requirements of mourning (and other) behavior. Still another explanation may be that women, being generally of lower status than men, are expected to take on the symbolic burden of distress and grief for the whole community. Finally, it should be pointed out that a lifetime of economic dependence on a man may lead women to experience the loss of a spouse more keenly than a man does. In the following lament from a widow among the Jivaro, the themes of dependency and loss are clearly mixed: "O my dear husband, why have you left me alone, why have you abandoned me? . . . Who will hereafter fell the trees for me and clear the ground to make the manioc and banana plantations, or help me with cleaning and tending the fields? Who will hereafter make a red-striped *tarachi* for me for the feasts, who will bring me game from the forest or the gaily colored birds which you used to shoot with your blowgun and your poisoned arrows? All this you did for me, but now you lie there mute and lifeless. . . . O, dear me, what will become of me?" (Rosenblatt et al., Note 4).

As has already been suggested, in many societies remarriage is expected and encouraged after a suitable mourning period. In these societies, there are various mourning ceremonies that have the effect of breaking ties with the dead spouse and thus encouraging remarriage. The most common of these are destroying or giving away the deceased's personal property, observing a taboo on the name of the deceased, changing the residence of the survivor, and changing feelings about the spouse through ghost fears. All these practices may be viewed as moving the spouse of the deceased to undertake new personal commitments more readily. Such rituals also make it easier for others to relate to the deceased's spouse in terms of new relationships.

Among the LoDagaa of West Africa, the funeral ritual is, above all, a time at which the social roles that the dead man, especially, played throughout his life are reallocated. Funeral ceremonies provide institutionalized procedures for other persons to take over these roles. This is done through the mechanism of funeral orations, accompanied by gifts. A person in a particular relationship to the deceased makes a speech about him, telling of his good qualities that were important in that relationship. The speaker then produces gifts of food and beer, which are offered to the dead man, but also to the person who is prepared to fill his place in the relationship. In these ceremonies the dead man's roles as husband and father, as friend and even lover, are handed over to others. The persons who accept the gifts also accept the responsibility of the roles, and of filling them not merely perfunctorily but satisfactorily.

It seems appropriate to end this chapter with the preceding account of the funeral customs of the LoDagaa, which contrast so strongly with our own. In the United States, the absence of funeral or mourning rituals that satisfactorily reintegrate the closest survivors of the deceased, especially widows, into new statuses and new social networks appears to underlie many of the emotional problems that death causes us. Almost without exception, studies have shown that widows, particularly, suffer increased isolation and feelings of depression at their husband's death. The LoDagaa, and other cultures like them, appear wiser than we in preparing for death and in developing their rituals, which—though they may seem outlandish and extreme to us—appear to be more than reasonably successful in meeting the needs of individuals and societies in their moments of greatest crisis.

REFERENCE NOTES

1. Huntington, R., & Metcalf, P. *Celebrations of death: The anthropology of mortuary ritual.* Cambridge: University of Cambridge Press, 1979, 29–30.
2. Freuchen, P. *Book of the Eskimo.* Greenwich, Conn.: Fawcett, 1961, p. 146.
3. Cannon, W. B. "Voodoo" death. *American Anthropologist*, 1942, *44*, 169–181.
4. Rosenblatt, P., Walsh, R., & Jackson, D. *Grief and mourning in cultural perspective.* New Haven, Conn.: HRAF Press, 1976, p. 12.

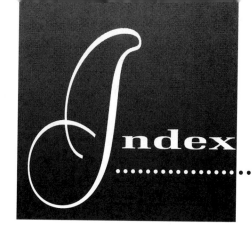

Index

A

Acceptance, 19
Acquired immunodificiency disease
 See AIDS
Adolescents
 perception of death, 14, 84
 suicide rates, 136
Advance directives, 125
African Americans and suicide, 137
Afterlife beliefs, 169–171
Age
 and grief reactions, 158
 and pain response, 70
 and suicide rates, 136–137
AIDS
 caregiver concerns, 112–114
 coping in, 107–108
 ethical issues, 115
 family and loved ones, 109–112
 financial issues, 106
 illnesses seen with, 105–106
 pain and determination, 108–109
 patient profiles, 104–105
 pregnancy and, 115–117
 routes and course of HIV infection, 101–103
 and social attitudes, 6, 9
 stigma of, 22, 59
 testing for, 101–102
 treatment, 106–107
Analgesia, patient-controlled, 94–95
Analgesics 74–75
 See also Pain
Anderson, Robert (writer), 155
Anencephaly, 122–124
Anger, 19, 154–155, 174
Anticipatory grief, 159–160
Anxiety, 16–18
Asian Americans and suicide, 138

Assessment
 of nurse's feelings, 31–32
 of pain, 72–73
 and suicide intervention, 144–148
Attitudes
 See also Cultural issues
 American social, 3–9
 and communication, 23–25
 individual and developmental, 13–26
 toward AIDS and HIV infection, 22–23
Australian Dreamtime belief, 169–170
Autonomy, 26
Awareness and disclosure, 57–58

B

Bargaining, 19
Bereavement, 153–166
 See also Grief
Biochemical theories of suicide, 141–142
Biofeedback, 73
Brain death, 121–124
Bureaucratic aspects of hospitals, 51

C

Camus, Albert, 139
Cancer, 20–22, 70
Cardiac disease, 20–22, 33
Caregivers
 attitudes toward dying children, 88
 attitudes toward pain, 75–76
 communication with children, 87–88
 concerns about AIDS, 112–114
 impact of suicide on, 149–150
CDC (Centers for Disease Control), 103–104
Children
 and AIDS, 116
 grief of parent, 159–160, 161–162

Children *continued*
  impact of suicide on, 148
  mourning rituals and, 173–174
  and pain response, 70
  perception of death, 13–14, 81–83
  and refusal of treatment, 126–127
Chinese cultural values, 25, 138
Collaborative care, 42–44
Communication
  awareness context, 57–58
  disclosure issues, 56–58
  with family, 34–36
  and jargon, 54
  nurse–physician, 42–45
  physician–patient, 38–42
  and social attitudes, 23–25
  with terminally ill children, 86–88
  with well children, 84–86
Connecticut Hospice, 67
Coping skills, 25–26, 91–92
Counseling, grief, 164–165
Crib death (SIDS), 97
Crile, George, 156
Crisis intervention, 144
Cruzan, Nancy, 124, 130–131
Cultural issues, 12–13, 71
  See also Attitudes
  afterlife, 169–171
  appropriate feelings, 174–175
  attitudes to pain, dying, and death, 171–172
  grief reactions, 172–173
  rituals, 176–181
  social status of deceased, 173–174
  suicide, 137–138, 175–176

D

Death: legal definition, 121–124
Death and dying
  See also Terminal illness
  American social attitudes, 3–9
  communication and cultural values, 23–25
  compared with sick role, 39
  coping with, 25–26, 91–92
  developmental influences and, 13–16
  fear and anxiety about, 16–18
  individual perceptions and attitudes, 13–25
  institutionalization of, 6–7
  mortality patterns, 5–6

  as process, 18–20
  societal perceptions and attitudes, 3–9, 56–57
  stigma and, 20–23
On Death and Dying (E. Kübler-Ross), 18–20
Death rates
  See Mortality
Denial, 19, 84
Depression, 145, 146
  See also Suicide
Despair, 155
Development and perception, 13–16
Disclosure
  See Communication
DNR (do not resuscitate) orders, 52, 59, 130
Dobu culture, 175
Doctors
  See Caregivers; Physicians
Durkheim, Emile, 139
Dying
  See Death and dying; Terminal illness
Dying trajectory, 18–20, 59–60

E

Economic issues, 52–53, 59, 106
Elderly
  See Older persons
Emotional involvement of nurse, 36–38
Ethical issues
  See also Legal issues
  in AIDS, 115
  definition of death, 121–124
  euthanasia, 127–132
  refusal of treatment, 124–127
Euthanasia
  active and passive, 127–128
  direct and indirect, 128
  legal issues, 129–131
  religious issues, 131–132
  voluntary and involuntary, 128–129
Extended-care facilities, 61

F

Families
  See also Support systems
  and disclosure, 57
  grandparents, 93–94
  nurse and, 34–36, 160–161

parents 89–92
  of persons with AIDS, 109–111
  role changes with death, 162–164
  siblings, 92–93
  suicide's effect on, 148
  of terminally ill children, 89–94
Fear
  of death, 16–18, 90–91
  of persons with AIDS, 110–111
Financial issues
  See Economic issues
Freud, Sigmund, 140–141
Funerals, 176–178
  See also Cultural issues; Grief

G

Gender
  and grief reactions, 158
  and pain response, 70
Germ theory, 49
Gikuyu society of Africa, 169
Grandparents
  See Families
Grief
  anticipatory, 159–160
  behavior in, 153–154
  caregivers' role, 160–161, 164–165
  cultural differences, 172–173
  pathological, 157–159
  phases of, 154–156
  symptomatology, 156–157
  types, 158
Grief counseling, 164–165
Group therapy, 92, 148

H

Harvard Medical School New Pathways
  program, 41
Hastings Center guidelines, 124
Health care providers
  See Caregivers; Nurses; Physicians
Hindi view of pain, 170
HIV infection
  See also AIDS
  routes and course of disease, 101–103
  stigma of, 22–23
  testing for, 101–102, 107
  transmissibility, 112–114

Home care, 60, 94–95
Hospice care
  in AIDS, 109, 114
  for children, 94–95
  history, 65–67
  and pain management, 69–77
    See also Pain
  in United States, 67–69
Hospice home health program, 68
Hospital hospice, 67–68
Hospitals
  See also Hospice
  alternatives to, 60–61
  and attitudes toward death, 6–7
  as bureaucracies, 50
  care versus cure, 53–55
  disclosure of information, 56–56
  history, 49–50
  impact of suicide on staff, 149–150
  influences on care level, 56–60
  and pain management, 76–77
  patient's role, 54–56
  role expectations, 54–54

I

Illness as Metaphor (S. Sontag), 21
Independent hospice, 68
Infants
  death of, 96–97
  perception of death, 82
Informed consent, 24
Institutionalization of death, 6–7, 76–77
Insurance
  See Third-party payment
Inuit (Eskimo) suicide, 175–176

J

Japanese social structure, 25
Japanese suicide rates, 138
Johnson, Earvin "Magic", 102–103

K

Kübler-Ross, Elisabeth, 8, 18–20, 67

L

Latinos and suicide, 137

Legal issues
    See also Ethical issues
  definition of death, 121–124
  euthanasia, 129–131
Lewis, C. S. (writer), 154–155
Lewis, Oscar (sociologist), 174
Life expectancy, 5–6
Lindemann, Erich (sociologist), 156

M

Media and social attitudes, 7–9, 82
Medical education, 40–41
Medicare/Medicaid
    See Third-party payment
Menninger, Karl, 141
Middle age, 15
Mortality
  from cardiovascular disease, 21
  changing patterns of, 5–6
Mourning, 153–166
    See also Grief

N

Narcotic drugs
    See Analgesia; Pain
Nerve blocks, 73–74
Nightingale, Florence, 49
"No code" orders, 52, 59, 130
Nurses
  attitudes toward terminal illness, 31–32
  communication with physician, 42–45
  and dying patient, 32–34
  emotional involvement of, 36–38
  and family unit, 34–36
Nursing homes, 61

O

Older persons
  perception of death, 15–16
  suicide rates, 136–137
On Death and Dying (Kübler-Ross), 18–20

P

Pain
  acute and chronic, 70

  in AIDS, 108–109
  analgesics in, 74–75
  assessment, 72–73
  caregivers' attitudes toward, 75–76
  control, 73–74
  cultural attitudes, 171–172
  perceptions of, 70–72
  Ten Commandments of, 77
Parents
    See Children; Families
Philosophical theories of suicide, 139
Physicians
  attitudes and communication, 38–40
  communication with nurses, 42–45
  medical school education, 40–42
Piaget, Jean (psychologist), 82–84
Pneumocystis carinii pneumonia, 102–103,
  105, 107
    See also AIDS
Pregnancy and AIDS, 115–116
Preventionist theory of suicide, 142–143
Process of dying, 18–20
Psychoanalytic theory of suicide, 140–141
Psychosocial aspects of death, 13–16

Q

Quinlan, Karen Ann, 129–130

R

Race and suicide rate, 137–138
Reevaluation counseling, 92
Refusal of treatment, 124–127
Reintegration, 156
Religion, and euthanasia, 131–132
    See also Cultural issues
Respect, 32–33
Rituals of death and mourning, 176–181
Role changes with death of spouse, 162–164
Role expectations, 39, 53–55

S

Saikewicz, Joseph, 125
Saunders, Cicely 8, 65–67
Self-help groups 92, 148
Serotonin and suicide, 141–142

Sex
> *See* Gender

Sexism, 52, 104–105

Sexuality and AIDS, 110

Shneidman, Edwin, 142, 148

Siblings
> *See* Families

Sick role, 39, 53–55

Sontag, Susan (writer), 21

Saint. Christopher's Hospice, 65–67

Stages of dying, 18–20

Stigma of dying, 20–22

Sudden infant death syndrome (SIDS), 97

Suicide
> *See also* Euthanasia
> age and, 136–137
> caregivers' response, 147–148
> cultural attitudes, 175–176
> gender issues, 138–139
> impact on survivors, 147
> prevention of, 143–147
> racial and cultural issues, 137–138
> rate of occurrence, 135–136
> theories of, 139–143

Suicide intervention, 146–148

Support systems, 25, 92, 111, 148

T

Talking
> *See* Communication

Television
> *See* Media

Terminal illness
> compared with sick role 39
> and helping professions, 31–45
> *See also* Caregivers; Nurses; Physicians

Third-party payment, 59, 69, 106, 115–116

Tikopia society, 170

Toddlers, 82–83

Touch therapy, 32–33

Trajectory of dying, 18–20, 59–60

Tuberculosis, 113–114

V

Values clarification, 32

Veach, Robert, 122

Voodoo, 176

W

Widows/widowers, 163–164
> *See also* Grief

Witchcraft, 176

Y

Young adults' perception of death, 14–15

3